Becoming with Care in Drug Treatment Services

Employing Deleuzo–Guattarian orientations to assemblage and feminist approaches to care, this book offers a critique of neoliberal approaches to recovery from drugs and alcohol, while collapsing the dualities of harm reduction and recovery.

This monograph empirically explores the practices of care emerging in two drug recovery services in Liverpool and Athens. Following the flows of the participants' desires, it argues that it is not the lack of the substance that holds the recovery assemblage together, but the production of connections that enhance a body's power of acting, constituting recovery a practice of collective care. The outcome of the analysis of the lived experiences of people in recovery is a call for the dismissal of policy as an intervention coming from outside, and its reconstitution as a practice produced inside the recovery assemblage.

Focusing on the value of the assemblage as a viable methodological, onto-logical and epistemological orientation for critical drug studies, this volume contributes to the sociology of health and illness and will appeal to students and researchers interested in fields such as Deleuzian Studies, Science and Technology Studies, Sociology and Social Policy, Drugs and Addiction, Public Health and Medical Anthropology.

Lena Theodoropoulou is Lecturer in Public Health at the University of Liverpool.

Routledge Studies in the Sociology of Health and Illness

For more information about this series, please visit: www.routledge.com/
Routledge-Studies-in-the-Sociology-of-Health-and-Illness/book-series/RSSHI

Becoming with Care in Drug Treatment Services

The Recovery Assemblage

Lena Theodoropoulou

Routledge
Taylor & Francis Group
LONDON AND NEW YORK

First published 2023
by Routledge
4 Park Square, Milton Park, Abingdon, Oxon OX14 4RN

and by Routledge
605 Third Avenue, New York, NY 10158

Routledge is an imprint of the Taylor & Francis Group, an informa business

© 2023 Lena Theodoropoulou

British Library Cataloguing-in-Publication Data
A catalogue record for this book is available from the British Library

Library of Congress Cataloging-in-Publication Data
Names: Theodoropoulou, Lena, author.
Title: Becoming with care in drug treatment services :
the recovery assemblage / Lena Theodoropoulou.
Description: First edition. | Milton Park, Abingdon, Oxon ;
New York, NY : Routledge, 2023. |
Series: Routledge studies in the sociology of health and illness |
Includes bibliographical references and index.
Identifiers: LCCN 2022022911 (print) | LCCN 2022022912 (ebook) |
ISBN 9780367760168 (hardback) | ISBN 9780367761240 (paperback) |
ISBN 9781003165613 (ebook)
Subjects: LCSH: Drug abuse–Treatment–Social aspects. |
Alcoholism–Treatment–Social aspects.
Classification: LCC RC564 .T499 2023 (print) |
LCC RC564 (ebook) | DDC 362.292/86–dc23/eng/20220722
LC record available at https://lccn.loc.gov/2022022911
LC ebook record available at https://lccn.loc.gov/2022022912

ISBN: 978-0-367-76016-8 (hbk)
ISBN: 978-0-367-76124-0 (pbk)
ISBN: 978-1-003-16561-3 (ebk)

DOI: 10.4324/9781003165613

Typeset in Times New Roman
by Newgen Publishing UK

For Elsa

Contents

Figures

Acknowledgements

Writing is a collective process and the content of this book has been directly and indirectly informed by many encounters.

This book wouldn't have been possible without the participation of service-users and workers of 18 ano and Genie in the Gutter. I'm indebted to all workers of both services for their trust, and for sharing their insightful experiences and knowledge of recovery and care. I'm especially grateful to the artist and art therapist Adam Mavropoulos, the first person to introduce me to the 'little planet' of 18 ano. His enthusiasm, unique approach and long-term experience of recovery and art therapy have informed my growing interest in the field. Special thanks to Dimitris Yfantis, head of research at 18 ano, for his encouragement when a long time ago I shared with him my desire to pursue a recovery-related PhD. Our discussions since then have provided me with an insight and knowledge that I wouldn't have gained otherwise. I am also indebted to Panayiotis Zaganiaris for accepting me at 18 ano's theatre group. Thanks to his endless energy and knowledge, every single group has been a unique learning experience.

The service-users of 18 ano and Genie in the Gutter that participated in this study will remain anonymous. I cannot however emphasise enough how much the life and story of each one of them matters. I'm extremely grateful to all of them for trusting me and supporting this project by making it their own. Although integrating all our discussions in one book wouldn't have been possible, our encounters have shaped my understanding of recovery, and subsequently hold a very special place in the development of the ideas presented in this book.

The research presented was undertaken as part of a PhD programme at the University of Liverpool, in the department of Sociology, Social Policy and Criminology. I'm grateful to my supervisors, Nicole Vitellone, Vicky Singleton and Karenza Moore, for their insightful, consistent and caring supervision. Their expertise has assisted me in the development of crucial aspects of this study. This book would not be what it is without Nicole Vitellone's support and our long-term collaboration. Nicole's collegiality and care exceeds all expectations, and I can't thank her enough for that.

I'm also grateful to colleagues and mentors who have informed my way of thinking. A special thanks to Ciara Kierans, Cameron Duff and Melanie Manchot. I would also like to thank colleagues from the Centre of Health, Medical and Environmental Humanities, University of Liverpool, and from the Contemporary Drug and Alcohol Studies programme at the University of the West of Scotland.

I'm thankful to the Economic and Social Research Council for financially supporting all aspects of my PhD, and to the Centre of Health, Medical and Environmental Humanities, University of Liverpool, for supporting the writing of this book.

Many thanks to the production team at Routledge and Lakshita Joshi. Some of the content of this book has been previously published and I'm grateful to the publishers for their permission to reproduce it:

Chapter 6: Theodoropoulou, L., 2021 'Describing recovery from drugs and alcohol: how "small" practices of care matter', *Qualitative Research*, Special issue on 'Doing Things with Description: politics, practice and the art of attentiveness', 21(3), 409–425.

Chapter 7: Theodoropoulou, L., 2020 'Connections built and broken: the ontologies of relapse', *International Journal of Drug Policy*, Special issue on 'The ontopolitics of drugs and drug policies', vol. 86.

Beyond the academic world, I am grateful for the friendship of many amazing people who have informed my way of being and thinking. In London, Liverpool and Athens, a massive thank you to you all, you know who you are. Special thanks to Filyra Vlastou, Maike Pötschulat and Laura Harris

I'm extremely lucky for growing up in a loving and supporting family. Many thanks to Neni Nikolaou and Tzimis Papoutsis. I'm grateful to Anna Papoutsi and Tania Papoutsi; growing up with them has shaped me in all sorts of ways. A lot of love and a massive thank you goes to my dad, Sakis Theodoropoulos, for his unconditional vote of trust in me and my choices. This book is dedicated to my mum, Elsa Nikolaou, for being an endless source of love, strength and inspiration throughout her life.

Introduction

Reclaiming recovery

'Recovery' is not a new term in the treatment of drug and alcohol use; from the 19th century onwards, it has acquired various different meanings and has been deployed to describe diverse treatment practices (Berridge, 2012). Accordingly, the term 'recovering subject' has accounted for various different relations between a person and a substance. People on opioid prescriptions, those in detoxification clinics and residential rehabilitation centres, as well as former users abstaining from illicit and prescribed drugs for specified or unspecified periods of time are talked about as recovering subjects (Frank, 2018; Nettleton, Neale and Pickering, 2013). These diverse 'identities' – shifting from heroin to methadone, from substance use to abstinence and from drug using subjectivities to recovering subjectivities – and the ways in which they come into being within the recovery space, have been the focus of attention of several research studies (Dahl, 2015; Fomiatti, Moore and Fraser, 2019; Hughes, 2007; McIntosh and McKeganey, 2000). In this book, my focus is on the practice of recovery as it emerges through the everyday encounters and connections enabled in two recovery services. Following the lived experiences of the service-users and workers of those services, I explore the flows of care that enhance the recovering body's capacity to affect and be affected. The emphasis is not on individual identities, but on collective becomings. The space of recovery is not presented as the 'solution' to a 'problem', but as a 'site of potentiality' (Zigon, 2019: 120), unfolded as a complex amalgam of human and non-human forces that opens up new life possibilities.

The current growing focus on the 'recovering subject' emerged as a critical response to the shift of many national policymaking strategies from harm reduction to the 'recovery model'. Critical accounts of this policy turn have adopted the Foucauldian lens of biopower and governmentality (Nettleton, Neale and Pickering, 2013), while others focus on a wider understanding of normality and sociality (Fomiatti, Moore and Fraser, 2019).[1] Current researchers and practitioners of recovery in Australia and the UK are increasingly reaching the agreement that recovery 'means more than abstinence or reduction in substance use, and should encompass improvements in other areas

DOI: 10.4324/9781003165613-1

of clients' lives, including housing, relationships, employment, participation and wellbeing' (Lancaster, 2017: 758; also see Dennis, Rhodes and Harris, 2020; McKay, 2017; Neale, Nettleton and Pickering, 2012; Neale et al., 2014; Theodoropoulou, Vitellone and Duff, 2022), while acknowledging the risk and resisting the implementation of 'a set of neoliberal assumptions about work, productivity and what it means to live a "contributing life"' (Lancaster, 2017: 758).

Overall, in theory and in practice, recovery has been primarily associated with prohibitionist models and neoliberal politics and ethics, leading to the question posed by Fomiatti, Moore and Fraser (2019: 536), of whether the concept of recovery is salvageable or should be abandoned. They suggest that contemporary health governance is underpinned by neoliberal premises that render it difficult to make recovery anew.

I argue that recovery should not be abandoned but reclaimed, and we can do so by staying with the trouble and complexity of recovery (Haraway, 1988) – that is, if we focus on how recovery is done in practice, rather than accept how it is framed in policy documents; if we challenge the dualism of harm reduction versus abstinence; if we draw on the lived experiences of people in recovery, then maybe the concept of recovery does not have to be abandoned, or even made anew. This task of reclaiming recovery requires that we reclaim policy too. I do so by challenging the notion that policy must emerge *outside* the practice of recovery and be subsequently implemented on those practices. Conversely, the object of this book is the *practice* of policy (Gill, Singleton and Waterton, 2017), as it emerges organically *inside* the recovery space, entangled with the becoming practices of care. By shifting our gaze to caring practices, and how policy emerges through them, the 'present' of recovery and how and why it matters can be seen otherwise: recovery in this book is not defined as the interruption of the relationship between a body and a substance, nor as the implementation of policy, but rather as a practice of care that grows organically within drug treatment services.

My commitment to sideline the neoliberal politics that equate recovery to abstinence and normality, and to reveal instead how daily recovery practices create a politics of worldbuilding (Zigon, 2019) does not derive from a 'neutral' position, but from my previous engagement with drug treatment services as an art therapist trainee and recovery worker. 'A politics of worldbuilding is a form of politics that seeks to allow potentiality to emerge as new possibilities for being-with, thus laying the onto-ethical grounds for new worlds' (Zigon, 2019: 13). Zigon encountered a politics of worldbuilding through the activism of people who use drugs, people who create communities of solidarity that make a 'living otherwise' possible. My first encounter with a politics of worldbuilding was in 2012, when I was training in art therapy at 18 ano, the Athens-based drug recovery centre I collaborated with for this research. In the financial and social crisis-struck Greece, 18 ano was at the time not just practising recovery, but a politics of worldbuilding, foregrounding solidarity as the force that renders a 'living otherwise' possible. Closely observing recovery practices that attempt to lay the grounds for new worlds, and at the same time following the construction of recovery as an essential aspect of drug strategies based on prohibition and the criminalisation of people who use drugs, raises the question 'to whom does "ethical" and "effective" treatment belong?' (Garcia, 2015: 3). Following the practices of two recovery services, in Athens and Liverpool, my aim is to show that 'ethical' and 'effective' treatment belongs to the service workers and the service-users who practise, challenge and change the meaning of recovery through their lived experiences. By holding this positionality, I do not argue that there is no space for critique of the practices that inform these services' treatment approaches. However, reflecting Gomart's (2004) stance, I believe that in these critical times in which austerity politics, applied internationally, prevail over the needs of those who ask for help, it is vital that as researchers, we stand with and actively trust and support the practices of those who craft recovery daily.

The two services I 'stand with' in this book are 18 ano and Genie in the Gutter. 18 ano, the service I conducted research with in Athens, is a two-year-long recovery programme structured in three stages. During the first stage, service-users are supported in their attempt to maintain abstinence from substances. Once this has been achieved, they move on to the second stage, which is residential and lasts for seven months. One to one and group psychotherapy as well as art groups are the main activities they engage with. Finally, the last stage is called 'social reintegration' and lasts for approximately one year. The aim is to support service-users in the development of connections with the community. With Genie in the Gutter[2] I had not worked with in the past, and I got to know the service's treatment practices while I was volunteering there as part of my fieldwork process for this study. Genie is a day recovery-focused service based in Liverpool city centre. Their aim is to support people who identify as addicted to drugs and alcohol to reduce their use or achieve abstinence.

The prerogative of this book is the exploration of novel ways to talk about recovery. How can we describe and make sense of the practices becoming in the recovery space? The process of recovery is emotionally intense, and one of the main challenges has been to capture this intensity, without resorting to emotive ways of talking about people's lives. I have chosen to address these complex connections by understanding the recovery space and process as an assemblage, in the Deleuzo–Guattarian sense of the term. Although I specifically focus on the practices emerging in 18 ano and Genie, I situate these practices within the wider field of the sociology of health and illness. Accounting for the affective relationships produced in the recovery space extends our understanding of drug using realities, of the desires invested in the recovery process, and of the ways in which societies fail those whose desires clash with dominant systems of thought and practice. Unpacking recovery as an assemblage has provided me with the vocabulary, the structure and the frame of thought needed to stay with its complexity. Unlike Foucauldian analyses, which primarily understand recovery as a practice of care of the self (Nettleton, Neale and Pickering, 2013: 177), the Deleuzo–Guattarian perspective has opened the way for the analysis of the recovery process as a practice of collective care (McLeod, 2017), through which the recovery subject is produced not as an individual but as a body whose happiness is entangled with its capacity to affect and be affected (Duff, 2014a). The recovery assemblage is where human and non-human components come together to enhance a body's capacity to act, and to support its desire of becoming-other. The structure and content of the book reflect the epistemological, methodological and empirical becoming of the recovering assemblage.

The first chapter, 'Engaging with drug research through a feminist technoscientific lens', focuses on the difficult and troublesome connections that empirical researchers engage with, critically discussed through the lens of feminist accounts on practices of care. Through my reading of this body of literature, I ask 'who do empirical researchers care for and how?' (de la Bellacasa, 2011) and 'what kind of exclusions does this way of caring produce?' (Martin, Myers and Viseu, 2015). I specifically address these questions by exploring the ways in which scholars (Bourgois, 1995; Bourgois and Schonberg, 2009) include and exclude connections traversing their participants' lives, and the position that they hold in their fields of research (Garcia, 2010, Gomart, 2004, Knight, 2015). I conclude that care, as it is practised in empirical research, needs to extend beyond the relationship between researchers and participants, to include all the connections and encounters that constitute our participants' drug using and recovering realities. The entanglement of drug use and recovery with policymaking (Fraser and valentine, 2008, Race, 2008, Zigon, 2011) is explored drawing on recent Science and Technology Studies (STS), which address the complex relationship between policy and care, and how these can be reconfigured together (Gill, Singleton and Waterton, 2017: 8). I argue that by following our participants' engagement with drug and alcohol services, and the practices of care produced in these spaces, we can start imagining *policy as a practice*, organically emerging through these encounters.

Following up on the argument that researching with care entails caring for the connections that traverse our participants' lives, in the second chapter I discuss how and why a Deleuzo–Guattarian system of thought enables us to do so. I specifically address the methodological pillars that traverse my analysis: the Deleuzo–Guattarian assemblage and its deployment in the empirical studies of Cameron Duff (2014a) and Kim McLeod (2017). For both Duff and McLeod, recovery does not happen to the individual; it is a collective process (McLeod, 2017) emerging through the material, affective and social assemblages that expand the body's power of acting (Duff, 2014a). Through their work, I navigated the complex space of recovery, focusing on the life possibilities becoming through the affective practices emerging in the recovery assemblage. The Deleuzo–Guattarian concept of the assemblage constitutes the core of my analysis, rendering possible the generation of affects and affective relations, becomings, desires, deterritorialisations and reterritorialisations. In this chapter, my engagement with these concepts for the unpacking of the recovery assemblage is outlined. Finally, I focus on the specific ways in which Deleuze and Guattari conceptualised drugs, and the methodological suggestions that they made for researchers and writers attempting to unfold the complexity of drug use. Although these are not suggestions widely deployed by scholars who discuss drug use through a Deleuzo–Guattarian prism, I argue that there is a methodological potential currently undervalued, especially in Deleuze's call to focus on 'causalities' and 'turning points'.

In the third chapter, I discuss how methods are deployed for the production of space-specific research, in and with the recovery assemblages in Liverpool and Athens. I specifically address methods as connection-building devices, producing, enhancing and accounting for the connections built between the two fieldsites, between the researcher and the services, and the researcher and the service-users. The research encounter was shaped and affected by various components like the space where one-to-one interviews took place and the relationship between the interviewer and the interviewee. Although initially the force that organised the structure of the interview was the substance, the stories narrated moved beyond it, accounting for all the connections built *around* the substance and how these matter, the desired becomings enabled and blocked through drug use. Accordingly, the encounters with recovery were not about the service-users' physical disengagement from substances, but about new connections, the life possibilities becoming through their engagement with services. The visual methods deployed rendered the connections produced during the interviews stronger, and the distance from the substance as the focus of attention larger. Drawing on McLeod's (2017) work with photography-based methods and deploying photovoice – giving the camera *and* the analytic voice to the participants – enhanced a shared commitment and the participants' sense of ownership of the project, producing not only another set of data, but also another way of building connections as a research method in itself.

The fourth chapter, 'Of other spaces: the birth of the heterotopia of recovery', addresses the historical identities of the recovery services involved in this study, as these emerged within specific cultural, political and policy-making contexts. Bringing together the Deleuzo–Guattarian assemblage with the Foucauldian 'other space' opens the way for the understanding of recovery's entanglement with the contexts within which it emerges, while simultaneously 'other' to them. In his text 'Of other spaces', Foucault (1986) argues that in our epoch, space takes for us the form of relations among sites. Among these sites, Foucault is interested in the ones that have the 'property of being in relation with all the other sites, but in such a way as to suspect, neutralize, or invent the set of relations that they happen to designate, mirror, or reflect' (Foucault, 1986: 25). He names these sites 'heterotopias'. Heterotopias are not idealised reflections of the societies through which their 'otherness' is established (Hetherington, 1997), but sources of 'ambivalence and uncertainty, thresholds that symbolically mark not only the boundaries of a society but its values and beliefs as well' (ibid: 49). Accordingly, the time of one's engagement with recovery signifies a rupture with the ways in which life was organised, in order to reflect on it and change it according to new desires that emerge. The heterotopia of recovery becomes in relation to other sites but also attempts to transform them by allowing ambiguity and uncertainty to be expressed. In this chapter, I address the histories of the recovery spaces I have been collaborating with in Athens and Liverpool, focusing on how these heterotopias came into being.

The fifth chapter, 'Becoming a drug user – becoming a service-user', follows the participants' first experiences of substance use, and their attempts to make sense of these past experiences, as recovering subjects in the present. Thinking with desire, the gaze is on the becoming-other, positioning not the desire *for* the substance in the focus of attention, but the investment of desire *through* the substance. Following the same line of thought, Deleuze's question on the causality of drugs is addressed. I then move on to discuss Deleuze's turning point, the moment when drug use shifts from a line of flight to a line of death (Deleuze and Guattari, 2004). Through the service-users' narratives, I argue that the turning point does not necessarily happen when one encounters a substance for the first time, but when this encounter is accounted for as a rupture in time, when drug use *makes sense* in a different way. This chapter also contributes to the literature accounting for the relationship between so-called dependent drug use and freedom. The empirical data produced addressing the participants' experiences of drug use as a daily practice demonstrate a shift of the drug from an agent of becoming-other to an obstacle that blocks flows of desire. Finally, I return to Deleuze's turning point, to account for one's shift from becoming a drug-user to becoming a service-user. Going beyond the often emotively deployed 'rock-bottom' experiences that initiate engagement with recovery services, I focus on service-users' encounters with care in drug-using environments, and the desires that these encounters mobilise.

The sixth chapter of this book closely follows the service-users' engagement with the material, affective and social assemblages of recovery, an analytical framework based on Duff's (2014a) analysis on recovery from mental illness. To account for the material recovery assemblage, I return to Foucault's heterotopology, to demonstrate how the recovery space is produced *differently*, as another, safe space, frequently juxtaposed to the 'outside'. The specific practices of 'turning up' for appointments and 'checking-in' with service-users are discussed as caring practices that contribute to the production of the territoriality and temporality of the recovery assemblage. Through small transformative gestures and the production of a mutual commitment between workers and service-users, the shift from drug using time to recovery time becomes possible, as the recovery space gradually becomes more attractive than the drug using one. The affective assemblage is unfolded through service-users' accounts and understandings of therapeutic boundaries, as well as through the generation of hope and the life possibilities that feeling 'hopeful' opens up. The aim is to trace the thresholds the body crosses, in its transformation with the recovery assemblage. The social assemblage is accounted for from both within the recovery space, but also as it extends beyond it. Extending beyond spaces of recovery, the recovery assemblage is not expected to simply enable the engagement of service-users with other assemblages, but to equip them for the struggles yet to come.

The chapter, 'Beyond the recovery assemblage', further problematises the encounter of the recovering subject with assemblages that extend beyond the recovery space, and explores the forces that build barriers blocking the flow of desire, forces the recovering subject is confronted with throughout, and especially after their disengagement from the recovery assemblage. Focusing on perceptions of employment, I render visible the clash between the desire to *work towards* something, as this is nurtured in the recovery assemblage, and the measurement of one's 'worth' based on their employment status. Through the empirical data produced, it is demonstrated how the desires of recovering service-users, the desire to 'slow down' and become connected, are in conflict with neoliberal systems of time. While the service-users' narratives provide an explicit understanding of the components that contribute to their wellbeing, in the assemblages where they are called to 'reintegrate', these components are not taken into consideration, hence putting the wellbeing of recovering subjects at risk. It is within this framework that 'relapse' is addressed. Following Deleuze's syntheses of time (1994), I argue that relapse might constitute an intrinsic component of one's process of becoming-well. However, in other cases, it might also be the outcome of a policy failure, of the rupture of the connections enhanced in the recovery assemblage.

The conclusion specifically focuses on policymaking practices. I draw examples of how the desire of services *to produce policies*, through their daily encounters with service-users and the practices of care provided, has been blocked. Finally, I argue that the dominant theoretical, methodological and empirical research finding that this empirical sociological study has produced is the need to dismiss policy as an intervention, and to reconstitute it as a practice. The practices of care unfolded in this book *are* policy in practice, demonstrating that what is missing is not more policy changes or reforms imposed on the services, but protective mechanisms that enable the practices of care becoming in the recovery assemblage, and support the becoming other of the recovering body beyond it.

Overall, this book is not an attempt to provide a manual on how recovery should be done, regardless of the social, political and cultural assemblages within which it becomes. Conversely, it is a biography of two specific recovery assemblages, as they emerged and developed their practices within concrete socialities, and as these were experienced and talked about by service-users and workers who were part of these assemblages at a specific time. I am not interested in providing an unconditional praise of recovery overall. It is only by looking at *specific* recovery practices that we can argue whether these lead to the reproduction of dominant moral systems or to a resistance to them, via a fresh 'evaluation of what bodies 'can do' in their encounters with one another' (Duff, 2014a: 153). This positionality is in line with the methodology deployed for the analysis of these assemblages. Foucault, in his preface to *Anti-Oedipus*, emphasised that it would be a mistake to read it as 'that much-heralded theory that finally encompasses everything, that finally totalizes and reassures, the one we are told "we need so badly" in our age of dispersion and specialization where "hope" is lacking' (Foucault, 1977: xii). Accordingly, I am not treating the work of Deleuze and Guattari as a methodological 'tool' that unlocks all doors and provides all the answers needed, but as a system of thought that can help us navigate the recovery assemblage in all its complexity, without getting lost.

Notes

1 For an extensive critical review of empirical research on recovery from drugs and alcohol, see Vitellone, Theodoropoulou and Manchot, 2022.
2 Referred to as 'Genie', from now on.

Chapter 1

Engaging with drug research through a feminist technoscientific lens

In this chapter, I engage with qualitative research on drug use and recovery, focusing on the difficult and troublesome connections that empirical research sometimes addresses and other times excludes. Thinking with feminist technoscientific scholars, I am interested in the configuration of caring connections between researchers and participants, and, subsequently, in whether and how these connections translate into engagements with policymaking practices. Drug using practices constitute the core of the difficult connections empirical researchers engage with, emerging among participants, between participants and researchers and between researchers and policymakers. What is often missing from this engagement is an alliance with the institutions and people positioned in-between drug users and the design of policy: the services and workers that sometimes apply and other times resist policy, through their daily practices. I attend to this omission by focusing on the lived experiences of people in recovery from drugs during their engagement with services. Doing so produces an engagement with policy in practice, and accounts for connections that extend beyond the encounter between a subject and a substance. These connections become visible when we shift our attention from drug using practices emerging in spaces of use, to caring practices emerging in spaces of recovery.

Recent Science and Technology Studies (STS) address the complex relationship between policy and care, and how these can be reconfigured together (Gill, Singleton and Waterton, 2017: 8). While recovery remains underexplored, policy, care and empirical research can be reconfigured together through a close exploration of recovery practices. Rephrasing Helen Keane (2002), I ask 'What's wrong with recovery?' Why is it difficult, unsettling and troublesome to talk about recovery and subsequently, which connections are neglected through the non-engagement with recovery practices?

Empirically and in practice, ethnography's aim is to care about difficult connections. Murphy (2015: 721) defines care as a commitment to be troubled, worried, sorrowed, uneasy and unsettled. Deploying this definition of care, I address the ways in which ethnographers care for their participants

DOI: 10.4324/9781003165613-2

through the commitment to make sense of the difficult connections traversing drug users' realities. I then discuss how the positionality of the researcher in the field affects the form that care takes, and shapes the knowledge produced.

Difficult connections: the response of drug ethnography

In his ethnographic account *In Search of Respect: Selling Crack in el Barrio*, Bourgois (1995) deploys Bourdieu's (1998) concept of 'cultural capital' to reveal the impenetrable barriers that separate the skilful East Harlem's crack dealers from legal employment. Bourgois simultaneously acknowledges the agency of his subjects by analysing their illegal activities as a – by no means ideal – way of resistance to classifications imposed on them. Bourgois's aim is to refrain from presenting drug dealers and street-level criminals as 'exotic others', and to place them instead 'into their rightful position within the mainstream U.S. society ... [To show that] they are 'made in America' (Bourgois, 1995: 26). Bourgois is also interested in the connection between drug using practices and individual responsibility. In *Search of Respect* (1995), his focus is on how his research subjects embody the responsibilities imposed on them:

> *They [crack dealers], like most people in the United States, firmly believe in individual responsibility. For the most part, they attribute their marginal living conditions to their own psychological or moral failings. They rarely blame society; individuals are always accountable.*
>
> (Bourgois, 1995: 54)

Bourgois is not interested in exploring whether his participants *are* responsible for their living conditions, but rather *why* they hold themselves accountable for failures that derive from structural social inequalities imposed on them. Bourgois's thinking opens up a new way for understanding social and policy failures that accompany drug users' lives. By making them the focus of attention, and *caring for* their life-stories and their attempts to move from the underground to the real economy, he unfolds the various ways in which drug users are excluded from formal economic structures.

In *Righteous Dopefiend* (Bourgois and Schonberg, 2009), the connection between the homeless drug users whose lives Bourgois and Schonberg follow and the social apparatuses in which they are expected to participate becomes more complex. This complexity derives from the association of political, financial, cultural and institutional forces with structural and personal abusive relationships that define homeless drug users' lives – described by the authors 'as lumpen abuse' (Bourgois and Schonberg, 2009: 16). By following this line of thought, Bourgois and Schonberg overcome the representation of drug users as one more excluded population and situate them within the current sociopolitical reality of the context they are researching. This approach brings to the surface a series of difficult connections to be accounted for. While the description of drug users as co-producers of the social constitutes them as active agents rather than passive victims of an unjust system, it also raises for the authors the question of the relationship between drug using realities and individual responsibility. By focusing on the agency of their participants, Bourgois and Schonberg argue that the abusive connections that dominate their lives have to be accounted for. Unlike *In Search of Respect*, where Bourgois was mainly concerned with the participants' difficulty to become part of the legal economy, in *Righteous Dopefiend* (2009), he attempts to makes sense of the complex relations between his participants, the coexistence of abuse and solidarity informing their experiences of drug use and homelessness.

The fundamental question Bourgois is attempting to address in his ethnography with Schonberg (2009) is 'How do we, as researchers, talk about troublesome subjects?' In auto-ethnography, this issue is negotiated through a reflexive analysis of narrated events (see, e.g., Hunter, 2018 and 2020). However, the gaze of the 'outsider' researcher is split between the ethical responsibility to address all aspects of participants' lives and the lack of theoretical and analytical tools to do so. My interest in Bourgois's work has to do with how empirical researchers choose which practices and connections to care for.

According to Martin, Myers and Viseu (2015), 'care is a selective mode of attention: it circumscribes and cherishes some things, lives, or phenomena as its objects. In the process, it excludes others' (627). Understanding care in this way is important for the comprehension of the exclusions that derive from researchers' choices (see also Lindén and Singleton, 2021). Following his commitment to render visible his participants' social isolation, Bourgois situates himself in sites where homelessness is enacted. His focus is on spaces created by the people he follows, and on the relationships that shape those spaces. Through the adoption of this ethnographic gaze, the connections of his participants with institutions and services, beyond sites of homelessness – hospitals, social services, harm reduction and recovery services – are sidelined, and the connections generated in those sites are excluded from his fieldwork and empirical analysis.

This positionality is also reflected in Bourgois and Schonberg's analysis of harm reduction practices. In their critique, harm reduction is seen as a means for the reproduction of a middle-class public health discourse that refuses to adjust to the constraints that accompany the 'lumpen subjectivities' of their ethnography (Bourgois and Schonberg, 2009: 106). What would be interesting to see as part of their analysis is a closer engagement with the harm reduction practices they criticise, and with the workers who deliver them. Bourgois and Schonberg's empirical and analytical object of research is the drug and the connections that its consumption produces. Spaces where the user gets disconnected from the drug fall outside their primary field of research. The connections happening *without* drug use are not accounted for.

In her account of addicted and pregnant women living in daily-rent hotels in San Francisco, Kelly Ray Knight (2015), ethnographer and student of Bourgois, situates herself differently. Knight does not follow the drug, but the thread of the addicted women's own narratives, carefully exploring the connections that derive from their accounts, and in so doing she provides a holistic account of *all* the apparatuses – medical, policymaking, social – that traverse these women's everyday lives. Knight manages to achieve her ethical commitment 'to write against an anthropology of easy enemies in which the tools of ethnographic engagement are wielded to attribute blame and produce affect in a manner that elides nuance and complexity' (Knight, 2015: 30). In so doing, Knight creates ruptures in the discourse of the worthy and unworthy poor, where the unworthy are held responsible for their suffering, while the worthy ones are seen with compassion (ibid.).

Ethics of care and the researcher's positionality

In her ethnographic account, *The Pastoral Clinic: Addiction and Dispossession along the Rio Grande* (2010), Angela Garcia provides a geography of addiction, taking into consideration the historical, cultural, political and social contexts that shape the identities of New Mexico's Española Valley drug users. In her sociocultural contextualisation of addiction, Garcia stays with the complexities of her research subjects, and in particular with the trouble of relapse. Relapse in her ethnography is not narrated as an event that happens to the individual, but as a collectively embedded practice that emerges from the social and political history of the geographical place her participants inhabit. Garcia therefore manages to challenge discourses of blame that discuss relapse as a failure of the individual. Instead, she foregrounds systemic failures, and how these affect the everyday lives of the drug users of Rio Grande. Garcia cares for her participants by extending her gaze to their social and political environments, providing a theoretical analysis that extends beyond the individual and focuses on the formation of collective subjectivities.

The object around which connections are built, broken and analysed is once more the drug. Garcia tells the history of Rio Grande *through the drug*, and produces it as the object that connects Rio Grande's past and present. Unlike Bourgois and Schonberg who were situated in spaces of drug use, Garcia's empirical 'base' is a detoxification clinic. It is here that she meets and then follows her participants to their personal spaces, explores their connections with the histories of the space they inhabit and attempts to make sense of their relapses through these connections. What would be interesting to see is Garcia's reflection on her own positionality, not only as a researcher but also as a worker at the detox clinic. Whilst she focuses on the development of her own emotional proximity with her participants, the connections that hold the detox clinic together are not accounted for. In situating herself in a recovery setting, Garcia refrains from talking about recovery practices, regarding recovery as an impossible task, focusing on the sufferings and abuses that traverse her participants' lives.

Like Bourgois and Garcia, Gomart's (2002) empirical focus is on a substance, the methadone, and the connections that derive from its administration at the 'Blue Clinic', a substitution clinic in Paris. While for Garcia the detox clinic is an extension of her connection with New Mexico, Gomart situates herself in the field of research differently. Gomart is interested in the specific connections made possible through the practices of care emerging in the Blue Clinic. Her attention is on building connections not only with participants but also with practices:

> *Rather than starting from an identification with drug users, I searched for 'colleagues' among care professionals and drug users who asked the same questions as myself. I would not assume they were* like *me; but I would allow that others pose questions with me … I 'followed the actors', to use an often quoted phrase of Latour's, in the sense that I sought to learn from them, staff and users at the Blue Clinic, how to set up the conditions of my competence.*
>
> (Gomart, 2004: 86, emphasis in original)

Being aware of her identity as a researcher, Gomart becomes part of the clinic she researches. By caring for, and taking seriously all actors involved in the specific setting, she acknowledges the service-users and workers of the clinic as allies in a shared struggle:

> *in the midst of this debate on methadone, where actors must take a position for or against each other, where funding can be won or lost because of a rumour or an academic article in a foreign language, I collude with the Blue Clinic team* and *clients.*
>
> (Gomart, 2004: 87, my emphasis)

Gomart's positionality in the field of research is also telling of the practices she chooses to care for. From a feminist technoscientific lens, care is a knowledge-making practice (Martin, Myers and Viseu, 2015: 627). De la Bellacasa, in her thinking with the work of Donna Haraway, argues that care is not an abstract expression of interest but comes with the responsibility of the researcher 'to ask critical questions about *who* will do the work of care, as well as *how* to do it and for *whom*' (de la Bellacasa, 2011: 91). In Garcia's work, the answers to these questions derive from her care for the connections between her participants' drug using realities and New Mexico's troublesome history. Garcia addresses collective caring through her call for 'watchfulness' *with* one another, meaning 'to offset forms of alienation that accompany addiction and to insist on the persistence of certain intimate ties' (Garcia, 2010: 182). Garcia's approach is interesting as it discusses 'watchfulness' as an ethics of community and a form of care, based on the creation of meaningful relationships. Through her call for watchfulness that transcends spaces of recovery and extends to all New Mexico's social encounters, Garcia stays faithful to her commitment to render visible the entanglement between drug use and New Mexico's history. Conversely, the knowledge that Gomart produces focuses on the connections that the substance creates *inside* the recovery space. Her practice of collective care is enacted by her active participation and alliance with all actors affected by these connections.

Kelly Ray Knight's (2015) ethnography on pregnant, addicted women in San Francisco is produced through a different caring gaze. As mentioned earlier, Knight's starting point for the unravelling of connections is not the drug, but San Francisco's daily rented hotels. Situating herself in these spaces, she follows all the human and non-human encounters taking place inside it, and extending beyond it. In her account, knowledge is produced by the – as much as possible – unmediated inclusion of voices, apparatuses and institutions that shape addicted women's lives, regular residents of daily rented hotels. Care is not talked about, but actively practised by taking seriously 'all the social actors who are called on to address pregnancy and addiction, including addicted, pregnant women, their care providers, and policy-makers' (Knight, 2015: 233). In this sense, the knowledge produced and by extension the care provided are based on the close examination and demonstration of the complexity of the addicted, pregnant women's lives.

The different ways in which ethnographies make sense of the entanglement between practices of care and knowledge production are further emphasised through Garcia's and Knight's encounter with the unsettling issue of maternal responsibility during their fieldwork. In the following extract, Garcia comments on the potential responsibility of one of her participants, Lisa – a drug user herself – for her daughter's death from an overdose. Garcia writes:

> *When she finally did speak of her own possible role in her daughter's death, she did so in terms of* not knowing *her daughter was in trouble or in pain. She would ask 'Why didn't I know?' … And each time I heard Lisa utter these words, I wanted to ask her, 'How could you* not *know?'*
>
> (Garcia, 2010: 180, emphasis in original)

In these field notes, Garcia is troubled by Lisa's claim that she 'didn't know' (that her daughter was in trouble). In Garcia's eyes, the drug is omnipresent. Throughout her ethnographic work, she follows heroin closely, explores the connections it builds and breaks, the relief it offers and the suffering it evokes. By situating heroin in New Mexico's social history, she also understands *why* it is there, why injecting drug use is such a common practice of Rio Grande's inhabitants. What she cannot account for is why her participants do not see what she sees. How can they be unaware of the power heroin holds in their lives, *how can they not know*?

By focusing on the connections deriving from a space, rather than a substance, Knight (2015) manages to address how the knowledge her participants hold is produced. The following quote from one of her interviews with a clinician shows how she carefully attends to the voices of all actors involved in her participants' lives. The discussion was about the regularly recorded inability of addicted women to maintain custody of their newborn children. The clinician said:

> *And when they lose [custody of] the kid, they are* devastated. *I mean really traumatized*, retraumatized. *And I want to say, 'Wait a minute, come on. You must have seen this coming?' But she didn't. She didn't see it coming. She didn't, really, know it was going to happen. Not before it did. I don't know if it is holding onto hope, or just the ability to compartmentalize the addiction from everything else that is going on.*

Knight's comment on the clinician's words:

> *And this clinician was right. She didn't [see it coming]. For many women, the present was imbued with future projections (the chance of motherhood, a future baby born tox-negative) and haunted by past ghosts (a traumatic childhood, years of addiction). These temporalities competed with the persistence of present needs: the next fix, a way to pay for one's hotel room, the next meal.*
>
> (Knight, 2015: 10, emphasis in original)

Knight then moves on to discuss the various temporalities that shape the complex lives of addicted, pregnant women. The knowledge produced derives from the care-full consideration of the women's narrative. The phrase 'I didn't know' is turned into a question for the researcher – what prevented her from being able to know? Such an approach becomes possible through the empirical distance from the substance that Knight takes. By holding this positionality, Knight attends not only to connections associated with drug use, but also to hopes, memories, perceptions of motherhood, desires, aspects of one's life that the drug might be part of.

Knight's approach derives not only from the way she situates herself while conducting empirical research, but also through the acknowledgement of the distance between hers and her participants' lives. Knight's acknowledgement of her proximity and disassociation from the addicted, pregnant women she encountered constitutes an example of critical practice of care (Martin, Myers and Viseu, 2015: 636): 'I was present *and* distant. And I always went home at the end of the day, which in my case was to a house I owned fifteen blocks and a world away from the daily-rent hotels' (Knight, 2015: 25, emphasis in original). Although presence at the spaces participants inhabit is important, the recognition of the distance between the researcher and the participants is necessary. Care for the practice of research and those involved in it is not just measured by the presence, but also by the acknowledgement of the distance between the researcher and the participants. How we measure distance matters. Is it measured based on where *we* are or where the participants are? In her work with people with dementia, Latimer (2018b) says that 'we have to consider that it may be "us" that are elsewhere. Us, with our projects and our futures who are really away' (846). It might be our daily realities that prevent us from understanding how the knowledge that participants hold is produced.

By acknowledging that her 'ethnographic role produced knowledge while offering very little in immediate amelioration of suffering' (2015: 29), Knight's question is not whether care can be conducted through ethnographic work but if ethnographic work can *also* enable certain forms of care (ibid: 25, my emphasis). Her answer is not related to the physical presence of the researcher in the field, but to what she does as the beholder of these people's truths, how she re-presents her participants' voices and raises awareness of the complexity of their everyday lives.

How to see from below, as Donna Haraway (1988) argues, is not an easy task. There 'lies a serious danger of romanticizing and/or appropriating the vision of the less powerful while claiming to see from their positions ... The standpoints of the subjugated are not "innocent" positions' (Haraway, 1988: 584). Following this line of thought, my question towards empirical drug research is whether by positioning the drug at the centre, blind spots are created, preventing us from fully engaging with certain forms of knowledge our participants hold. What exclusions are produced when the drug stands as the main protagonist, and specifically how are caring 'others', like services and workers, excluded in this process?

Practices of policy and practices of care

Exploring the exclusions deriving from the choices of research subjects and the positionality of researchers in the field provides an insight into how ethnographers and other empirical researchers engage with policymaking practices. In problematising the relationship between policy and drug research, and in identifying the inclusions and exclusions produced through this connection, I argue that a shift of attention from the drug as a protagonist to the drug as a carrier of desire enhances our understanding of our participants' lives. In this process, the researcher's engagement with all human and non-human components of drug users' lives is required. Such components are harm reduction policies and recovery services and practices. These are spaces where policymaking as an external force is enacted or resisted. They are also spaces where policy can be understood differently, as a force emerging in practice through the connections that hold these spaces together. In order to shift the way in which we engage with and imagine policy, a closer engagement between researchers, drug services and workers is needed. Instead of adjusting findings to policy models, I argue for a policy that grows organically through the practices of care in place. Foregrounding the everyday interactions of the practitioners in the field, and the mechanisms they mobilise to care for each other and for the users of their services, it becomes the researcher's responsibility to closely attend to those mechanisms and enable their comprehension as a way to do policy in practice.

Fraser and valentine (2008) position the administration of methadone and the services that regulate it in a neoliberal context. They are interested in how methadone maintenance treatment (MMT) offers insights 'into the contemporary tensions and contradictions entailed in the production of the proper law-abiding, autonomous, responsibilised, "stable" subject of liberal society' (Fraser and valentine, 2008: 2). The 'experts' however remain present and in control of the methadone dosage. Through this professional regulation, the stereotype of the 'untrustworthy' addict is reproduced. Fraser and valentine argue that MMT services constitute spaces standing in-between legality and illegality, responsibilisation and regulation, blame and trust. Although they do not specifically engage with policymaking, their analysis highlights how MMT affects the bodies of drug using subjects *and* service-workers. They discuss how the professionalisation of services does not leave any space for caring practices. Conversely, it renders the workers of those services regulators responsible for policing drug users' bodies rather than carers responsible for the service-users' wellbeing. The description of this shift is highly important for the understanding of care as a force that does not follow a linear route – from the professional to the service-user – but is disseminated and shared in non-linear ways. In this context, practices of care not only refer to the users of services but also equally refer to the *workers* of those services, called to adjust their practices according to policy recommendations and instructions.

In drugs research, drug recovery programmes have also been explored as spaces of normalisation, where the deviant drug using subjectivity is transformed into a public health individual. Unlike the majority of ethnographic work, which focuses on active drug users and their social environments, Zigon (2011) has explored the lives and experiences of *recovering* drug users in post-Soviet Russia. In his ethnography *HIV is God's Blessing: Rehabilitating Morality in Neoliberal Russia*, Zigon makes an interesting connection between biopower and morality. He finds that the church-run recovery programme where he conducted his ethnographic research unwittingly produces subjectivities for a new regime of biopower:

> *responsibility has become the hegemonic moral virtue that any good neo-liberal subject must come to embody. By responsibility I mean an obligation to and for oneself as well as an Other, which is enacted by means of disciplined self-vigilance. Responsibility, then, is a dispositional attitude*

> *that enacts social relations by means of a hyper-self-aware individual who is*
> *able to stand outside of and be within those very relations at the same time.*
> (Zigon, 2011: 13)

For Zigon, responsibility in this neoliberal sense is one of the fundamental imperatives for the accomplishment of the 'normal' life the church-run programme prepares its residents for. The question of care from and to one another is sidelined by the disciplined vigilance of the self and others, aiming not at each other's wellbeing but at the establishment and maintenance of a normalising moral system. In Zigon's analysis, the workers of the service, in their attempt to support the recovery process and care for the service-users, become an inherent part of a policy framework that renders discipline as a condition for the provision of care.

Another example of ethnography's commitment to stay with recovery's complexity is Angela Garcia's ethnographic exploration of the practice of recovery in Mexico City's 'anexos' (2015), where she further exposes policy's inability to grasp the complexity, as well as the 'dark side' of care. The anexos are informal and unregulated drug treatment settings that 'utilize a form of violence *as* care to treat addiction' (Garcia, 2015: 1, emphasis in original). Participation is usually coercive, and 'therapeutic violence' is deployed as 'a mode of personal salvation and communitarian survival' (ibid: 4). Garcia is not interested in subjecting the anexos practices to moral scrutiny, but in exposing *how* violence becomes an integral part of drug treatment in the specific sociopolitical context, and what the anexos recovery practices 'reveal about the nature of recovery in a context where poverty, drugs, and violence are existential realities' (Garcia, 2015: 2). In so doing, Garcia exposes care's ambivalence, as a practice neither good nor bad, but entangled with historical, political and social contexts (Theodoropoulou, Vitellone and Duff, 2022). Through the description of care's ambivalent provision, Garcia reveals policy's inability to create formal recovery settings that take into consideration the complex existential realities of Mexico's drug using population.

Going back to harm reduction, an attempt to think policy by focusing on its practice can be found in Race's (2008) call for a non-moralised approach to care. Race sees in the application of harm reduction a potential of what he calls the great refusal, meaning 'the refusal to make public care *conditional* on adherence to moralized norms around abstinence' (Race, 2008: 418, emphasis in original). According to Race, this becomes achievable through *practical care*, provided irrespectively of categories of deviance that lead to the exclusion of certain groups. In other words, what he suggests is an ethics of care that does not focus on the identities of the subjects but on the *practices* and *conditions* within which their drug use emerges. Race's approach is an example of the ways in which research can engage with policymaking, without excluding or standing against those expected to apply policy through their everyday practices.

The main issue that the above studies bring to attention is the inability of policy as a force emerging outside spaces of treatment, to enhance the practices of care emerging in these spaces. The work of Fraser and valentine (2008) touches this subject through the description of service-workers whose safety – but not necessarily their wellbeing too – is guaranteed only when their contact with service-users is mediated by physical barriers. Zigon (2011) demonstrates how the quest for normality can dominate the way care is provided, and Garcia (2015) exposes the complex, dark side of care. Race (2008), from another perspective, focuses on specific and pragmatic policy recommendations and challenges the dominant policy discourses by dismissing the question of moral practices as unable to grasp drug users' realities. These empirical studies reveal policy as a force that limits care and blocks '… the conditions of possibility through which practitioners and patients alike are participants in world making, and through which care becomes an emergent property of their alignment not their division' (Latimer, 2018a: 389).

Reviewing the relationship between research and policy, Campbell and Shaw (2008) argue for the deconstruction of policy. They call for the disengagement of the researcher from the policymaker, as the complexity of the realities of research subjects cannot be captured through policy-dominated systems of thought, unless reduced to prefabricated subjectivities. Campbell and Shaw believe that by engaging with policy, researchers consent to the absorption of critical ethnographic practices by the state and their reshape into a regulatory regime (Campbell and Shaw, 2008: 691). Although this positionality is useful for the problematisation of policymaking overall, in what follows, I return to STS scholars to explore the potentiality, not of the deconstruction, but of a different engagement with policy. I argue that our focus should not be on whether or not academic researchers should engage with public policy debates, but on *how* we engage with it. Following Murphy's call for unsettled care (2015) and looking at policy as practice (Gill, Singleton and Waterton, 2017), I ask whether policy should also be unsettled, and eventually reoriented towards enabling organically developed practices of care, rather than attempting to design them outside the spaces from where they are practised.

In their paper '*Critical compassion: Affect, discretion and policy – care relations*', Singleton and Mee (2017) address practices of care in theory and practice. They demonstrate the various positive and negative affects the term 'compassionate care' carries, depending on whether it emerges in (policy) theory or everyday practice. Taking as a starting point new policy interventions that aim at the promotion of compassionate care, they expose 'care's darker side: its lack of innocence and the violence committed in its name' (Martin, Myers and Viseu, 2015: 627). Singleton and Mee (2017) juxtapose the policy-driven codification and quantification of compassion, making practitioners feel that they are constantly under surveillance (131), to collective practices of compassionate care that practitioners embody in an attempt to care for each other. They argue that the specific policies they engaged with 'do not adequately acknowledge relationality, affect and discretionary tinkering as aspects of compassion' (Singleton and Mee, 2017: 144). They conclude that

> *the challenge for future work is to bring care and policy together analytic-*
> *ally, methodologically and practically, perhaps by understanding both as*
> *practices of selective attention towards specific objects of care and simul-*
> *taneously away from others.*

(ibid: 145)

This commitment to explore how 'the relationship between care and policy is shaped in locations of practice' (Gill, Singleton and Waterton, 2017: 5) provides an alternative way of thinking policymaking practices in the field of drug use and recovery. With regard to harm reduction, for example, it would imply a shift from its understanding as a biomedical technology bound to specific policy instructions, towards its analysis as a form of care, as it is practised in specific locations. The work of Emilie Gomart (2002, 2004) is indicative of how practices of care can be encountered anywhere, as long as there is a dynamic and liberating set of relations in place. Gomart (2002) argues that the administration of methadone does not necessarily produce neoliberal systems of operation, since the relationship between the user and the drug differs according to the specific settings where it comes into being. Gomart believes that substitution is not a by default oppressive apparatus, but a space that can contribute to the production of another subjectivity.

In the following chapters, I draw on Singleton and Mee's (2017) analysis of (compassionate) care in practice, and Martin, Myers and Viseu's (2015) call for remaining unsettled with care. My aim is to talk about care as a force that connects all actors involved in drug use and recovery, to explore 'how policy and care might be reconfigured together' (Gill, Singleton and Waterton, 2017: 8), and to start imagining how an organically developed drug policy practice would look. Expanding Singleton and Mee's (2017) call for work that brings care and policy together analytically, methodologically and practically, I argue that the empirical is equally important in our engagement with care and policy, and I demonstrate how empirical research and attentiveness to the lived experiences of service-users and service-workers can reconfigure policy in practice.

The desire for an assemblage of care

This selective engagement with empirical qualitative drug research has followed and problematised the positioning of the drug as the centre of attention. Care is selective (Martin, Myers and Viseu, 2015), and by choosing to care for the connections produced through the drug, exclusions and blind spots are inevitably created. Such an exclusion is an empirical engagement with drug treatment practices. As discussed earlier in this chapter, some of the researchers who situated themselves in spaces of drug treatment and recovery refrained from specifically engaging with those practices.

Talking about recovery is difficult because it requires a shift of our attention from the drug to other connections. This does not imply a replacement of the drug with another object. The problem with recovery is that it does not provide another object or dominant force to stabilise our focus, to indicate from where connections start. It is complex and confusing, a difficult connection on its own account. However, it is due to this inherent complexity that recovery can be the way to talk about neglected difficult connections – connections produced in the absence rather than the presence of the drug. Engaging with recovery requires an acknowledgement that the object of our research is slippery, and the connections we have to account for are difficult. They do not follow linear narratives and making sense of them is a troublesome task. They do though open up a way to think about policy differently. Thinking with recovery is a way to shift from drug research that looks at policy in abstract, to an engagement with policy in practice.

The Deleuzo–Guattarian concept of the assemblage – and the system of thought developed by the two philosophers overall – is produced *as a way* to talk about difficult connections. It is most certainly not simplifying them – thinking with Deleuze and Guattari is a difficult connection on its own – but accompanies us in our attempts to make sense of complex connections as we stand within them. Through Deleuze and Guattari, and while becoming with the recovery assemblage, I trouble the connection between policy and care. Recovery is the space where difficult connections happen, where the practice of connecting takes place through the flows of care traversing it. It is these flows of care that I discuss as the becoming of policy in practice, policy emerging inside the space of drug treatment.

Thinking with Deleuze and Guattari has shifted my attention from the drug to the 'efforts [of drug users] to exceed and escape forms of knowledge and power and to express desires that might be world altering' (Biehl and Locke, 2010: 317). By embracing complexity as a collective issue, shared by researchers *and* research subjects, the aim is to produce knowledge that attributes 'to the people we study the kinds of complexities we acknowledge in ourselves' (Biehl and Locke, 2010: 317). Locke, in his attempt to make sense of the forces that drive the staff of the social services in post-war Sarajevo, identifies a *desire for care* (Biehl and Locke, 2010: 334, my emphasis). In this chapter, I have discussed care from a technoscientific feminist lens. In what follows, I stay with this epistemological framework for my engagement with the caring practices that traverse the recovery assemblage, and I mobilise desire as the link between Deleuzo–Guattarian systems of thought and feminist perspectives on care. While STS scholars have systematically deployed Actor–Network theory (ANT), a Deleuzo–Guattarian methodology has enabled me to stay with my intention to position the consumption of substances and their effects in the background of my analysis, and to primarily focus on the desired becomings that the drug (or the lack of it) is expected to render possible. It is thus not the object, and the networks that extend from it, but the desire of becoming-other, and the assemblages that its investment produces, that drives my analysis.

The shift of attention from the drug to desired connections is an attempt to imagine how Latimer's (2018a) call for a shift from heroic to small-scale aspects of healthcare can be put in action, in addiction and recovery research. By focusing on practices of care as assemblages in which persons, social processes and things interact, we 'can also reveal how "neglected things" are as important occasions for care as any of the more heroic aspects of healthcare' (Latimer, 2018a: 385).

Feminist technoscience studies follow an approach that 'interrogates both the harmful and nurturing aspects of care' (Gill, Singleton and Waterton, 2017: 9). My interest is in the 'nurturing aspects of care', in specific caring practices encountered in the localities where they are produced. Taking seriously Singleton and Mee's 'challenge for future work to bring care and policy together analytically, methodologically and practically' (2017: 145), my primary concern is to demonstrate how these 'nurturing' caring practices also constitute policy practices that can lead to organically developed policies, attentive to the service-users' desire for care. In the chapter that follows, I outline how a Deleuzo–Guattarian approach enables a close exploration of those practices.

Chapter 2

Thinking recovery with the Deleuzo–Guattarian assemblage

In the majority of the English-speaking world (US, UK and Australia), two contrasting approaches dominate the academic and policy discourse on drug use and treatment: the harm reduction approach, understood as the 'progressive' approach to drug use that promotes safe ways of using to ameliorate quality of life, and the recovery model that promotes abstinence and criminalisation of drug use. Ground-breaking research in the sociology and anthropology of drug use has been critical of the ways harm reduction is practised (Bourgois, 2000; Fraser and valentine, 2008; Walmsley, 2012). Furthermore, scholars have contributed to the amelioration of the practice of harm reduction by paying attention to the relations between the human and non-human components that constitute the everyday realities of drug users (Dennis, 2019; Race, 2008; Vitellone, 2017). This emphasis on harm reduction has produced insightful knowledge for the understanding and improvement of drug realities. Conversely, the concept of recovery has been claimed by conservative discourses, which in turn has meant that recovery practices have not been adequately explored. This book attends to this omission. It argues that there are multiple ways to do recovery, and thus generalising statements that classify it as 'good' or 'bad' do not attend to its complexities. Practices of recovery can lead to the reproduction of dominant moral systems or to a resistance to them, and it is only through a close examination of specific recovery assemblages, and by taking the voices of everyone involved seriously, that we can start approaching the question of recovery.

The focus here is on the sociology of recovery, people in recovery, their lived experiences and their trajectories from drug using to recovering subjectivities. The aim is to develop alternative methods that take the experiences of people in recovery as the central source of knowledge production. These voices constitute a source of knowledge production in three crucial ways: firstly, they provide an insight into drug using practices that draws on recent lived experience. Secondly, they offer insights on the *practice* of drug treatment, the relationships produced and reproduced within the recovery space and its limitations within specific sociopolitical contexts. Thirdly, *the way* that people

DOI: 10.4324/9781003165613-3

in recovery talk about drug use and recovery offers insights on the societal elements of the *system* of recovery, the post-recovery subjectivities that it produces, and how these reflect the particularities of the context within which they emerge.

Situating people in recovery as the focus of attention does not constitute an attempt to undermine the voices of active drug users. By no means is it implied that people in recovery hold a certain 'truth' or knowledge that drug users are unable to see. The voices of those engaging with recovery services expand our knowledge of drug realities by accounting for both the desire to use drugs *and* the desire to stop using. The emphasis on the recovering subject, in its becoming from a drug user to a service-user, constitutes an attempt 'to understand people in a different kind of temporality – in between, in flux and transition – as they endure and try to escape constraints and articulate new systems of perception and action' (Biehl and Locke, 2010: 336). By dwelling *in the meantime* of this shifting identity, we produce a knowledge that matters in the moment of its formulation (ibid.).

My overall aim is to reclaim recovery and the politics associated with it from conservatism, neo-liberalism and overall moralistic systems of thought and to propose in practice a sociology of recovery, where the question of care and its practice is prioritised over the dilemma between harm reduction and abstinence. Drawing on empirical research in Greece and the UK, I argue that a close examination of recovery practices, their meanings and applications has a lot to offer to the struggle against the criminalisation and medicalisation of the drug using population. This approach provides another reading of recovery, as a practice and ethics of care that develops organically through the encounters enabled in each service.

Why Deleuze and Guattari

In the previous chapter, I drew on feminist perspectives of care to call for a shift of the research gaze in the sociology of drug use. I argued that getting to know and care for participants requires attentiveness to the connections becoming beyond the participant-researcher relationship. Through the exploration of two specific recovery sites, I engage with these support networks in a *positive* way. By positive I do not mean uncritical, but committed to follow, unpack, render visible and potentially expand the caring practices already in place.

Deleuze and Guattari, throughout their common and individual writings, focused on the human and non-human connections that traverse all aspects of life, and on the affects and possibilities that these connections render possible, or block. While 'more-than-human' ways of knowing have a long history in Indigenous ontology, epistemology, axiology and ethology (Bignall and Rigney, 2019), Deleuze and Guattari's writings emerge from within a commitment of Western philosophy to confront its own anthropocentric tradition. Their way of thinking life as an amalgam of forces, desires and territorialisations challenges the existence of an individual who thinks and acts in isolation. Instead, through their writings, subjects are fluid, always becoming through human and non-human encounters. This way of thinking inspired me to explore the encounters that potentially expand life possibilities in the recovery space *and* offered me the way to do so. While maintaining the participants' lived experiences as the main source of knowledge production, deploying a Deleuzo–Guattarian methodology enables us to follow the non-linear, complex threads of their desires, as these become through their encounter with the recovery assemblage. The decision to approach the recovery space through the Deleuzo–Guattarian assemblage emerged while doing fieldwork and experiencing the recovery process. Through my encounters with services and their users, I understood the process of recovery as never fixed but always becoming. By following the becomings, desires, affective relations and collective experiences, as these unfold in the recovery space, the significance of 'good' caring practices emerged as the pillar that holds all these forces together and enhances the assemblage's power to act.

In the existing literature on alcohol and other drugs (AOD), there is a significant body of work that mobilises the assemblage as well as other Deleuzian concepts to talk about drug and alcohol use (Bøhling, 2014, 2015, 2017; Dennis, 2016; Dilkes-Frayne, 2014; Dilkes-Frayne and Duff, 2017; Duff, 2014a, 2014b; Farrugia, 2015; Fitzgerald, 1998, 2010; Malins, 2004). Yet it has not been explicitly mobilised as a methodology for the exploration of recovery from AOD.[1] This literature is informative of the ways Deleuzo–Guattarian theories can be deployed while researching AOD in order to critically explore the context of drug and alcohol use (Bøhling, 2014; Duff, 2014a, 2014b), desire and pleasure as affect (Bøhling, 2017; Fitzgerald, 1998, 2010), the transformations and striations of the drug assemblage (Malins, 2004) and drug use as an event (Dennis, 2016; Dilkes-Frayne, 2014), and has contributed significantly to the enhancement of our understanding of drug realities. However, throughout my empirical research with people in recovery and the services they engage with, it has been studies on mental health, and specifically Kim McLeod's '*Wellbeing Machine*' (2017) and Cameron Duff's work on recovery from mental illness (2014a), that have enabled me to make sense of recovery practices. The deployment of these studies in order to talk about recovery from drugs does not imply an identification of drug use with mental illness. Following a Deleuzian way of thinking, I'm not interested in the classification and entrapment of subjects in moral categories like 'mentally ill' or 'drug dependent', but rather on the exploration of spaces where the relations, affects and events produced enhance the body's power of acting.

Therefore, the reasons for my choice to methodologically draw on Deleuzo–Guattarian studies on mental health are, firstly that the sociology of drug use has focused on the practices of active drug users, with the aim to inform harm reduction practices that better respond to the realities of the drug using population. My research has been on spaces of recovery from drugs and alcohol rather than on drug using environments. Unlike the drug assemblage, where the sociality produced is based on practices that primarily concern the drug using population, in the drug recovery assemblage the emphasis is on the encounters that enhance a body's capacity to act, as these become in the recovery space. Additionally, in the drug assemblage, the main non-human component the assemblage emerges from is the drug itself, the substance that is being consumed and the sociality produced around it. In the drug recovery assemblage on the other hand, it is not the substance anymore but its *absence* that holds the components of the assemblage together. It can be argued that although the drug is not *physically* present, this does not mean that it is *absent*, and that the drug assemblage continues to exist in different ways. The fact though that it is not being consumed *within* the recovery assemblage shifts the focus of attention to the production of affective relations that are not held together by the substance. Drawing on studies where the substance is not present has shifted my attention to the desired becoming-others, occasionally enabled or blocked by a substance, but not dependent on it.

Secondly, the theoretical roots of 18 ano, the recovery service I collaborated with in Athens for this project, lay on the British democratic psychiatry movement (see Cooper, 1967; Kooyman, 2001; Rawlings and Yates, 2001), the anti-psychiatric movement of the 1960s, put in practice by Franco Basaglia in Italy (Foot, 2015), and the institutional psychotherapy movement developed by Jean Oury and Felix Guattari in France (Genosko, 2009), at the psychiatric hospital La Borde. Although these movements were born in mental health institutions, they inspired an abstinence-based drug recovery model that due to its political characteristics stands against prohibition, criminalisation and normalisation. This model originated and was applied in France by the psychiatrist Claude Olievenstein, founder of the drug recovery centre Marmottan (Olievenstein, 1977), who defined addiction as the result of a triple encounter between a substance, a personality and a particular sociocultural moment. The treatment approach of 18 ano is inspired by Marmottan, and stands by Olievenstein's definition of addiction. This strong theoretical link between recovery and radical approaches to mental health and illness drawing from these movements also extends to the ways in which service-users and workers practise and experience the complex process of recovery. The issues addressed in McLeod's (2017) *Wellbeing Machine*, and Duff's account on recovery from mental illness in *Assemblages of Health* (2014a) helped me to stay with the complexity of the participants' narratives and, later on, also informed my research with participants from Genie, the service I worked with in Liverpool. Overall, the questions raised when addressing health and illness from a Deleuzian perspective are significant in our research with people using or recovering from drugs. The question, for example, '[h]ow might matters of health and illness be assessed in terms of flows and becomings rather than stable bodies and subjects?' (Andrews and Duff, 2019: 128), extends to the analysis of the lived experiences of drug using bodies, as well as to the shifting becomings of people in recovery.

Finally, the third reason I am drawing on the mental health assemblage is also associated with my fieldwork experience: in both Greece and the UK, I conducted fieldwork with services that have the particularity of accepting people who aside from identifying their drug use as problematic have also been diagnosed with a mental health illness. This is not common practice when it comes to drug and alcohol services (Matsa, 2007), but it responds to a growing need, as the number of drug users who live with a mental health condition (usually referred to as comorbidity or dual diagnosis) keeps increasing (Kelly and Daley, 2013; Matsa, 2018; Ross and Peselow, 2012, also reported by workers of 18 ano and Genie in the Gutter during our interviews). According to Genie's keyworker, this segregation in the treatment of mental illness and addiction creates confusion for the service-users:

> My previous experience, it was simply recovery, so anyone with other issues, mental health issues, anything else going on for them, was set aside and separate it out, so one person can be going to six different places out here. One person can come here and we'll try and deal with the six different things, so that's a difference in itself … Certainly when I'm observing the guys [service-users], a lot of them are not sure what's actually going on for them. They're confused around am I an addict? Is it mental health? Is it this? It's probably a combination of all, but what order do we deal with them in?

Therefore, an exploration of the recovery assemblage as one that not only addresses drug use but also enables connections that holistically enhance their service-users' wellbeing is more relevant than ever. In what follows, I address how Cameron Duff's *Assemblages of Health* (2014a) and Kim McLeod's *Wellbeing Machine* (2017) bring Deleuze into the sociology of health and illness, and how they specifically inform the methodological framework and structure of my analysis.

Assemblages of recovery and wellbeing

In *Assemblages of Health*, Duff explores 'the prospects of a posthuman account of health and illness, along with the value of such an account for research innovation in the health and social sciences' (2014a: 2). He mobilizes Deleuze's transcendental empiricism 'as a discrete methodology, capable of inspiring research designs more sensitive to "what we are doing"' (ibid: 26). In this context, the 'real experience' is understood in terms of the assemblage and the empirical explanation of how such assemblages are composed in distinctive events, affects and relations (ibid: 51).

As part of his empirical exploration of the assemblages of health, Duff accounts for the assemblage in recovery from mental illness, focusing on the therapeutic role of the community and social inclusion in supporting and promoting recovery. Recovery for Duff does not *happen to* individuals but emerges through a process – the process of 'becoming well', an *event* where an array of human and non-human bodies, forces, affects and relations are active (ibid: 94, emphasis in original). Duff is primarily interested in the 'actual experience' of social inclusion involved in the *production of recovery* in specific territories or milieus (ibid: 100). He identifies three assemblages of health that enable the emergence of recovery from mental illness: the material, affective and social assemblage.

The *material assemblage* refers to two articulations. The first one 'involves the selection and combination of "raw materials" out of which discrete territories are composed' (Duff, 2014a: 103), unique to each geological, biological or social entity. The second articulation establishes the function, meaning, purpose or form of the territory effected in the first articulation. However, none of these articulations are ever completed or fixed. They constitute a *movement towards stabilisation*, according to the historical, political, social and economic forces applied to, or expressed through them, rather than the final achievement of this state (ibid: 104, emphasis in original).

Accordingly, in my analysis I do not regard the recovery assemblage as a stable and fixed 'thing', but as 'the *process* of making and unmaking the thing' (Jackson and Mazzei, 2013: 262, emphasis in original). Through the accounts of service-users and the practices of care in place, I explore how the physical and symbolic territory of the recovery assemblage is produced, and how territory is claimed in the connections becoming in the recovery assemblage (ibid.). I specifically focus on how the discrete territory of the recovery assemblage is composed as a space of transition where the recovering subjects are enabled to restructure themselves in a way that extends their capacity to affect and be affected.

The *affective assemblage*: Affect describes an array of feeling states and equally constitutes 'the body's "power of acting"; its unique capacity to affect (and be affected) by the world of bodies and things that it encounters' (Duff, 2014a: 106). Within the social, positive affects become possible, like the ones associated with the experience of hope, where hope is always a belief in 'something more', a belief in that which has 'not yet become' (Anderson, 2006: 733–735). According to Duff, hope is fundamental in recovery from mental illness, as it affects the entire assemblage, investing it with greater scope in its power of acting (2014a: 107).

In the affective recovery assemblage, the territory of recovery is the transitional space where the becoming of the recovering body becomes possible, the space that allows for the 'generation of affective resources like hope, confidence or excitement to happen' (Duff, 2014a: 106). Becoming safe, becoming hopeful and negotiating boundaries are the affective practices deriving from the accounts of the service-users, enabling the development of new capacities and connections that enhance a body's power of acting, within the recovery space and beyond.

The *social assemblage*: Duff understands recovery 'as a *qualitative transformation in the assemblages that express the recovering body*' (2014a: 102, emphasis in original). This qualitative transformation becomes possible through the mobilisation of forces by which the social is enacted, including the '*desires* which conjoin bodies (human and non-human) in "social interaction"; the *affects* generated in such interactions … the *beliefs* that galvanise practical action in "social contexts" … as well as the *power relations* involved in efforts to regulate the conduct of the varied bodies assembled in the social mass' (ibid.). The assemblage of these social competences as they unfold in the recovery assemblage establishes diverse relations and actions that extend beyond and to other assemblages where these bodies operate (ibid.). Therefore, social inclusion and the cultivation of social ties are fundamental for the recovery from mental illness, as they enhance the body's capacity to act, to cross boundaries and constraints and to affect and be affected by various assemblages.

Duff is primarily interested in qualitative transformations as these become in various social assemblages and extend to others where a body operates, increasing its capacity to act. In this book, the focus is on *both* the sociality that emerges *within* the specific territory of the recovery assemblage (defined as an 'other' space that is affected by, but simultaneously different from the 'outside' that surrounds it), *and* the transformations of the other assemblages where recovering bodies operate. I initially account for the social body that emerges within the territoriality of recovery, specifically addressing the collective inhabitation of the recovery space as one of transition, and the affective relations and connections that emerge in the recovery and art groups. Drawing on service-users' accounts, it becomes apparent that the becoming-other emerging from the affective practices produced in the recovery assemblage *desires* to extend beyond it, to other assemblages. It is not a time and space-specific becoming, but 'a potential for action, a dispositional orientation to the world' (Duff, 2014a: 44). It is within this frame of thought that I discuss the encounters between recovering bodies and other assemblages, focusing on how the desire of becoming-other is claimed, negotiated and occasionally blocked, in its attempt to affect and be affected by other assemblages.

Kim McLeod (2017), in her empirical study of wellbeing, challenges the biomedical diagnosis of depression that is looking for symptoms, and calls for an investigation of the conditions and bodily encounters that lead to the formation of destratified assemblages. Overall, the *Wellbeing Machine* 'indicates how a series of *modulating* assemblages is necessary for lines of flight to be part of everyday life, in a manageable, sustainable way' (2017: 150, emphasis in original). McLeod is interested in how wellbeing is produced through the processes of everyday life (ibid: 3), focusing not only on processes of becoming-well but also on how wellbeing is informed by interactions and encounters that could be described as negative or destratified. Through the expansion of understandings about how wellbeing is mediated and the disassociation of states of illbeing with pathology, McLeod's work rethinks wellbeing 'in ways that do not blame individuals if they are not able to act, plan, and, make the correct choices toward improving their wellbeing' (ibid: 5). Mobilising Deleuze and Guattari's concept of the assemblage, she shifts the attention from the individual to the collective body (ibid: 15) and explores how 'illbeing, suffering and sad passions are in part generative, essential to the ongoing modulation of the *Wellbeing Machine*, and the possibility of emergent wellbeing' (ibid: 154).

This approach of wellbeing, as a process that emerges through encounters and interactions that do not follow a linear, becoming-well path, but are entangled with negative experiences and destratifications, has informed the analysis of the service-users' first encounter with a substance, as well as their subsequent engagement with recovery services. Following this methodological framework, 'becoming a user' is not pathologised; it is not a self-destructive act, a prevalence of illbeing over wellbeing, but an expression of a – potentially destratified – desire of becoming-well. Accordingly, 'becoming a service-user' is not an unconditional embracement of a 'healthy way of being', as health is understood by dominant and normative systems of thought, but an expression of the desire to work against practices that in the past have blocked a body's becoming-well.

McLeod's '*Wellbeing Machine* is made up of four assemblages which represent different affective capacities and different responses to the challenges of everyday life experienced by people with depression' (McLeod, 2017: 3): the Becoming-Depressed assemblage is described as a stratified assemblage, as it encompasses the desire for organisation, social agency and an active self. It provides a way of understanding pain and suffering as an illness requiring chemical treatment, 'works towards the stabilisation of all the institutions associated with depression' (ibid: 66) and follows the anti-depressant object 'as a connective resource for the formation of the organised collective body' (ibid: 65). The Becoming-Authentic assemblage forms as a response to the Becoming-Depressed assemblage and follows the human and non-human elements that contribute to the ongoing improvement of the participants' mental health. It includes lines of deterritorialisation and stratified relations, as positive affects like vitality, optimism and pleasure become possible, accompanied though by limitations, constraints and interrupted lines of flight (ibid: 97–99). 'The collective desire of this assemblage is for an enlivened self who can transform to a limited extent' (ibid: 98). The Becoming-Indeterminate assemblage comes as a response to those limits. This assemblage has an increased capacity to form relations to the outside, defined thus by its processes of deterritorialisation (ibid: 102). The affective flow is increased, and the emergent subject is not unified but rather in transition. 'The desire of this assemblage is to be able to collect-ively move across contexts and for the degree of transformations this affords' (ibid: 122). Finally, the Becoming-Destratified assemblage is about affective states of despair and immobilisation, encounters between assemblages that lead to destratifications (ibid: 127). 'The force of this assemblage, its power of acting or capacity to be affected, is only reactive and the affects that inhabit the Becoming-Destratified assemblage are only passive, and include the intensely-felt affective states of suffering and pain' (ibid: 147). In the 'Becoming-destratified' chapter of the *Wellbeing Machine*, McLeod follows her participants' lines of flight that turned into lines of destruction. In doing so, she empirically demonstrates illbeing as 'enduring, generative and neces-sary for wellbeing' (ibid: 167) and how suffering is an essential element in the dynamic experience of health, with the 'crack' being incorporated as an element in the machine' (ibid: 154).

The main difference between Duff's and McLeod's methodologies is the exclusion for the first and inclusion for the latter of illbeing, as a fundamental component of the 'becoming-well' process. Duff is primarily interested in the positive affects that take place in the recovery assemblage and argues that 'an ethics of recovery should ... take health itself, or the means of a body's becoming strong, reasonable and free, as its primary goal or substance' (Duff, 2014a: 190). Although he does not specifically argue that negative affects do not contribute to the becoming-well, he does not focus on their entanglement. He is interested in how forms of expression within specific assemblages are read, leading to perceptions of illbeing and wellbeing, based on the events through which an assemblage is encountered (Andrews and Duff, 2019: 125). McLeod (2017) on the other hand understands illbeing as essential for the emergence of wellbeing. For her, wellbeing is not the outcome of a process where the positive affects gradually prevail over the negative ones. It is the slow production of a solid construction that can handle suffering and pain without falling apart, in the same way that it can sustain happiness and positivity.

Despite this difference, both authors challenge 'conventional thinking about health, where the individual human body is typically regarded as the sole agent involved in the activity of health promotion' (Duff, 2014a: 105). Through the deployment of Deleuze and Guattari's concept of the assem-blage, they build a theoretical and empirical argument for the accomplishment of wellbeing as a collective process (McLeod) and the exploration of recovery as an event that does not happen to the individual but emerges through the material, social and affective assemblages that expand the body's power of acting (Duff). Instead of focusing on the symptoms of mental illness, they are interested in how people reconstruct themselves as part of and in relation to the socialities they inhabit. It is this line of thought that I am expanding to include the drug recovery assemblage, as an encounter of human and non-human components that expands the recovering body's power of acting. The aim of the drug recovery assemblage is the production of a sociality where the substance is *not needed* anymore as it is replaced by affective relationships that contribute to new becomings. It is this process of becoming-well within a new emerging sociality where research on mental health meets the drug recovery assemblage. Within this transitional space, a body's increasing capacity to act and be affected gradually emerges, extending beyond the drug recovery assemblage, to all other assemblages within which it operates.

McLeod and Duff are primarily interested in recovery and wellbeing within the community and in their participants' private environments. The focus of this book is initially on the service-users' desire of becoming-other, as this is negotiated within the territoriality of the recovery assemblage, and then extending to other assemblages where recovering subjects operate. I'm interested in exploring the organisation of the recovery space as an assemblage itself, and the ways in which this assemblage functions as an enabling space (Duff, 2011) for the emergence of wellbeing. Following McLeod and Duff in going beyond symptoms and behaviours, the past actions and future plans of the recovering bodies are not treated as evidence or indicators of what is expected of these bodies. The focus is on how experiences of illbeing and wellbeing are brought together in the recovery assemblage through the narratives of service-users, and on how these experiences are re-embodied and renegotiated through caring practices and the enablement of affective relations. Each drug recovery assemblage forms its own sociality, not in isolation but one that affects and is affected by the sociality within which it emerges. It constitutes a temporal, transitional and safe space enabling and defined by the affective relations that emerge within it. It is thus an open system where various 'becomings' take place and deterritorialisations are possible.

The Deleuzo–Guattarian assemblage and other concepts

In the next few pages, I provide an outline of my understanding of the Deleuzo–Guattarian assemblage, as well as of the other concepts (affect, becoming, desire and territorialisation) mobilised by the two philosophers and deployed for the description of the recovery assemblage.

Assemblages

There is not one way to talk about the assemblage. A fixed definition that encompasses all its potential uses would not be possible. Its own creators, Deleuze and Guattari, have complicated it by giving it half a dozen different definitions, with each one of them connecting the concept to a separate aspect of their philosophy (DeLanda, 2016: 1). This is reflected on DeLanda's (2016) provision of a systematic overview of the assemblage theory through a series of case studies that prove the concept's omnipresence and thus its potential for infinite applications: '... assemblages are everywhere, multiplying in every direction, some more viscous and changing at slower speeds, some more fluid and impermanent, coming into being almost as fast as they disappear' (DeLanda, 2016: 7).

In regard to the definitions of the assemblage given by Deleuze and Guattari, I stay with one of the first concept's descriptions[2] as it appears in *A Thousand Plateaus* (2004). According to the two philosophers, the assemblage is tetravalent, composed of a horizontal and a vertical axis, where both these axes comprise two segments. Horizontally, we encounter 'the *machinic assemblage* of bodies, of actions and passions, an intermingling of bodies reacting to one another' (Deleuze and Guattari, 2004: 97–98, emphasis in original). This is the content, the *pragmatic system* of the assemblage. On the other side of the horizontal axis, we encounter 'a *collective assemblage of enunciation*, of acts and statements, of incorporeal transformations attributed to bodies (ibid: 98, emphasis in original), the expression or *semiotic system* of the assemblage. The assemblage allows for a new relation to emerge between content and expression: 'the statements or expressions express *incorporeal transformations* that are "attributed" as such (properties) to bodies or contents' (ibid: 555, emphasis in original). Following this outline of the horizontal axis of the assemblage, the content, or *pragmatic system* of the recovery assemblage is composed of the bodies that inhabit it: the service-users and members of staff. On the other side of the horizontal axis, we encounter the daily practices of the assemblage, the recovery group, for example, the collective assemblage of enunciation where its expression comes into being.

The vertical axis of the assemblage is constituted by '*territorial sides*, or reterritorialized sides, which stabilize it, and *cutting edges of deterritorialization*, which carry it away' (Deleuze and Guattari, 2004: 98, emphasis in original). Territoriality and deterritorialisation are inseparable aspects of the assemblage.

> *Deterritorialization is the movement by which 'one' leaves the territory. It is the operation of the line of flight. It can be negative when overlaid by a compensatory reterritorialization obscuring the line of flight, or positive when it prevails over the reterriotorializations.*
>
> (ibid: 559)

The deterritorialisations and reterritorialisations of the recovery assemblage will be addressed in relation to the desires of the service-users as these become in its horizontal axis. I will demonstrate how the practices of care produced within the recovery space extend to other assemblages. The service-users' desire of becoming-other goes beyond their encounters with substances and their engagement with the recovery assemblage. Their accounts suggest another way of being in the world, another way of relating with all the other assemblages they inhabit. It is this potential, becoming possible in the recovery assemblage and extending beyond it that I understand as deterritorialisation. Conversely, reterritorialisation refers to forces, institutions and systems of thought that block deterritorisalisations.

Following this outline of the content, expression and territorial sides of the assemblage, DeLanda identifies four characteristics that traverse all assemblages:

> *1) Assemblages have a fully contingent historical identity, and each of them is therefore an* individual entity *... 2) Assemblages are always composed of heterogeneous components ... To properly apply the concept of assemblage to real cases we need to include, in addition to persons, the material and symbolic artefacts that compose communities and organisations ... 3) Assemblages can become component part of other assemblages ... 4) Assemblages emerge from the interactions between their parts, but once an assemblage is in place it immediately starts acting as a source of limitations and opportunities for its components.*
>
> (DeLanda, 2016: 19–21, emphasis in original)

These characteristics are present in the formation and operation of the recovery assemblage. The first one is addressed in the chapter 'Of other spaces: the birth of the heterotopia of recovery', where the historical identity of each one of the collaborating recovery services and the heterogeneous components that hold them together are discussed. The second of DeLanda's characteristics, the inclusion of the material and symbolic artefacts that compose communities, traverses all aspects of the analysis of the recovery assemblage. In regard to the third characteristic, in the introduction it was stated that this is not an attempt to provide an overall position on how recovery should be done. This positionality derives from the acknowledgement that the two recovery assemblages unfolded in this account constitute two individual entities, and accordingly, their practices are addressed in relation to their specific historical identities. At the same time, they are also part of various other assemblages: of the individual lives of the bodies that constitute them, of the wider socialities within which they emerge, of a national system of thought on recovery and further on, of a recovery assemblage that transcends borders and specific practices. Finally, the fourth characteristic is also addressed throughout the analysis, and specifically through the affective relations enabled by the negotiation of boundaries within the recovery space, and the deterritorialisations that these affective relations enhance.

Overall, the complexity of the assemblage is entangled with its omnipresence, with the fact that assemblages are able to account for infinite forms and shapes of encounters between human and non-human components. By staying with this complexity, my aim has been to accordingly stay with the complexity of the recovery space.

Affect and affective relations

Deleuze draws his definition of affect from Spinoza and his understanding of the body in terms of its capacity for *affecting* or being *affected*. According to Spinoza,

> *[t]hese are not two different capacities – they always go together. When you affect something, you are at the same time opening yourself up to being affected in turn, and in a slightly different way than you might have been the moment before. You have made a transition, however slight. You have stepped over a threshold. Affect is this passing of a threshold, seen from the point of view of the change in capacity.*
>
> (Massumi, 2002: 212)

Following Massumi's account of affect in the writings of Deleuze and Spinoza, affect and accordingly the affective relations enabled in the recovery assemblage refer to (1) the smaller or bigger transitions of a body in order to become part of and to sustain its presence in the assemblage, (2) the transitions that the collective body (all the individual bodies acting in coordination when driven by the same desire) of the assemblage allows to happen and (3) the slow transition of the assemblage itself, of its content and expression.

These three modes of transition do not happen separately; they are not different capacities, but transition together, passing thresholds and changing the assemblage's capacity to act. '[A]ll assemblages are only temporary accomplishments' (Andrews and Duff, 2019: 125), 'contingent and shifting interrelations among "segments" – institutions, powers, practices, desires – that constantly, simultaneously construct, entrench, and disaggregate their own constraints and oppressions' (Biehl and Locke, 2010: 323). It is through the affective relations that traverse it that this constant mobility of the assemblage is achieved. In the recovery assemblage, this temporality and fluidity are unfolded through the small shifts enabled through consistent caring practices. It is the daily gestures, a desire for care shared by all bodies, which constitute the recovery assemblage that increases a body's capacity to affect and be affected.

Becoming

> *it is not enough to simply observe that assemblages exist; we must attend, as Deleuze and Guattari originally urged, to the ways these configurations are constantly constructed, undone and redone by the desires and becomings of actual people – caught up in the messiness, the desperation and aspiration, of life in idiosyncratic milieus.*
>
> (Biehl and Locke, 2010: 337)

As stated by Biehl and Locke, just acknowledging an assemblage's exist-ence and observing it does nothing in regard to the understanding of the affective relations that hold it together. It is the desires and becomings of *actual people*, the *messiness* of life itself that constitutes the study of the assemblage much more than a theoretical exercise. The assemblage is never stable, but temporary, always in transition. It is through the term 'becoming' that Deleuze indicates this constant process of change in assemblages (McLeod, 2017: 39). Becoming, as Deleuze saw it, does not refer to a pro-cess, to a movement *towards* a stable state of being. Conversely, becoming *is* an ultimate existential stage itself, 'in which life is simply immanent and open to new relations – camaraderie – and trajectories' (Biehl and Locke, 2010: 317). In that sense,

> one does not become Man, insofar as man presents himself as a dominant form of expression that claims to impose itself on all matter, whereas woman, animal, or molecule always has a component of flight that escapes its own formalization ... To become is not to attain a form (identification, imitation, Mimesis) but to find the zone of proximity, indiscernibility, or indifferentiation where one can no longer be distinguished from a woman, an animal, or a molecule ... Becoming is always 'between' or 'among'.
>
> (Deleuze, 1998: 1–2, emphasis in original)

It is through the unfolding becomings that the narratives of the service-users in this book are accounted for. Starting from the time that one was becoming a drug user, the desires of becoming loved, becoming part of and becoming care-free are unpacked. Moving on to their engagement with recovery ser-vices, the becomings enabled through the affective relations that traverse the recovery assemblage are positioned in the focus of attention. Finally, the desired becomings that extend to other assemblages are explored. All these becomings are never stable. They escape concrete formalisations. They are not dominant forms of expression imposed on one's whole existence, fixed and settled identities, but fields to be explored, potential existential stages enabled by small transitions, by a body's increasing capacity to affect and be affected.

The practices discussed in this book are considered 'good' practices of care. However, care entails a dark side that needs to be taken into consideration. How do we make the distinction though, between 'good' and 'bad' practices, 'good' and 'bad' assemblages, becomings and desires? From a Spinozian point of view, moving in an ethical direction does not entail the attachment of 'positive or negative values to actions based on a characterisation or classifi-cation of them according to a pre-set system of judgment. It means assessing what kind of potential they tap into and express' (Massumi, 2002: 217). Within this ethical framework, the care practised in the recovery assemblage is regarded as 'good', based on the potential it taps into, and the enhancement of a body's capacity to act in ways that enable its desire to flow. As Massumi argues, 'good' and 'evil' are not intrinsic in practices or terms, but entangled with the becomings they enable:

> *The ethical value of an action is what it brings out* in *the situation,* for *its transformation, how it breaks sociality open. Ethics is about how we inhabit uncertainty together … Basically the 'good' is affectively defined as what brings maximum potential and connection to the situation. It is defined in terms of becoming.*
>
> (Massumi, 2002: 218, emphasis in original)

I argue that this is exactly what the *specific* recovery assemblages do. Their actions and practices are 'ethical' because they break sociality open *collectively*. The actors of the recovery assemblage inhabit the uncertainty of where desire will take them *together*, and it is through the connections enabled in the assemblage that they revisit past becomings, negotiate the present ones and imagine the future.

Finally, 'we must recognize the thresholds where liberating flights and creative actions can become deadly rather than vital forms of experimentation, opening up not to new webs of care and empathy but to systemic disconnection. Becoming is not always heroic' (Biehl and Locke, 2010: 336). For Deleuze and Guattari, there is a dead end in the becoming of a drug user, a line of flight that turns into a line of death. This is addressed through the accounts of the service-users in the chapter, 'Becoming a drug user – becoming a service-user'. Deploying McLeod's (2017) methods, I argue that a classification between 'good' and 'bad' becomings does not do justice to the complexities of the lived experiences of drug users, as experiences of illbeing are enduring, generative and necessary for wellbeing to happen (McLeod, 2017: 167).

Desire

Anti-Oedipus (1977), the first collective work of Deleuze and Guattari, is about desire. Foucault, in his preface to the book asks '[h]ow does one introduce desire into thought, into discourse, into action?' (Foucault, 1977: xii). Deleuze's and Guattari's response is that desire *becomes together* with the material reality of social production (1977: 30). There is no social production without desire, and accordingly, there is no desire standing in isolation, outside a machine or assemblage:

> *The first distinguishing feature of the theory of desire outlined in Anti-Oedipus (1977) is its positivity: desire is understood as a primary active force rather than as a reactive response to unfulfilled needs. Desire is productive in the sense that it produces real connections, investments and*

intensive states within and between bodies ... Deleuze and Guattari's theory of desire is constructivist in the sense that desire always requires a machine or assemblage.

(Patton, 2000: 70)

This understanding of desire differs significantly from the Freudian notion of desire 'as something that people possess and are perhaps possessed with ... Rather, desire [for Deleuze and Guattari] is something that intersects people, bodies and sociocultural realities. Desire is produced and present everywhere in life as an active life force' (Oksanen, 2013: 60). It is not a force imposed upon subjectivities, but one that renders becoming possible by cracking through apparently rigid social fields (Biehl and Locke, 2010: 323). In the recovery assemblage, '[i]t is the collective desire for difference that motivates activity' (McLeod, 2017: 16). The bodies assembled share the desire of becoming other, and through the affective relations enabled in the assemblage, they explore this desired becoming collectively.

The work of both services I collaborated with (18 ano drawing primarily on psychotherapeutic approaches, and Genie on more empirically produced understandings of the social needs of service-users) was very much focused on enabling people to shift their assemblages in ways that their capacities of acting were enhanced rather than diminished. This was achieved by producing the recovery assemblage in such a way that the desires of service-users were not blocked but enabled to flow. I follow this flow, to conclude that the desires driving one in becoming a drug user are not fundamentally different from the desires that lead one's becoming a service-user. There are no 'good' and 'bad' desires, but flows of desire enabled, and flows of desire blocked. Accordingly, the affective relations produced in the recovery assemblage do not change one's desire, but attend to the service-users' desire for care and connection. Finally, I argue that these caring practices produce a collective desire that 'can break open alternative pathways' (Biehl and Locke, 2010: 318), extending beyond the recovery assemblage.

Territorialisation (deterritorialisation and reterritorialisation)

Territorialisation as a force happens within the social, and 'provides an explanatory framework for how the forces of the social impinge on individuals or cultures, from the stratification of class, gender and ethnicity through to the construction of subjectivities' (Fox, 2002: 353). The distinction between reterritorialisation and deterritorialisation refers to whether territorialisation functions like a barrier or a border that blocks flows of desire (reterritorialization), or whether it breaks down such barriers (deterritorialisation) (Oksanen, 2013).

According to Deleuze and Guattari, '[p]eople are the continual subjects of deterritorialization and reterritorialization as their [bodies] are inscribed by the forces of the social' (Fox, 2002: 346). In the recovery assemblage, deterritorialisation is addressed as both momentary and inconsequential, as well as substantial and life-changing, a line of flight that carries the body 'into unimagined realms of possibility and becoming-other' (Fox, 2002: 354). The affective relations within the recovery assemblage enable small shifts and transitions of a body, gradually enabling the formulation of new connections and increasing its capacity to act. This process potentially leads to bigger, life-changing transitions, which render the desire of becoming-other possible. This desire extends beyond the recovery assemblage, affecting the other assemblages it comes in contact with.

For Deleuze and Guattari, the state is the assemblage of reterritorialisation par excellence, the one that effectuates 'the overcoding machine within given limits and under given conditions' (Deleuze and Guattari, 2004: 246). Through the analysis of the recovery assemblage, desire is decoded, invested in new ways that enhance a body's capacity to act. Conversely, I also discuss the ways in which dominant systems of thought recode this deterritorialised flow of desire, in its attempt to extend beyond the recovery assemblage. The state is present through these dominant systems of thought, through policy-making practices, perceptions on employment, worthiness and overall ways of being within the social. It acts as a reterritorialising force that limits the shape and form that flows of desire might take; it overcodes it in ways that can potentially block it and interrupt the deteritorrialisations becoming within the recovery assemblage.

However, it would be an oversimplification to classify deterritorilisation as solely positive, and reterritorialisation as an only negative force. What Deleuze and Guattari refer to as 'dependent' drug use, for example, is talked about as a negative deterriotorialisation, as a line of flight that fails to connect with other lines, turns into destruction and eventually becomes a line of death (2004: 253).

Deleuze and Guattari on drugs

Seen through the eyes of a critical reader today, the two philosophers' writings on drugs are unquestionably problematic. Deleuze and Guattari only understood drugs in their extremes: either as a destratified line of flight that becomes a line of death or as an encounter that takes the body's power of acting beyond imagination. For Deleuze, drug use becomes 'suicidal' the moment that dependence comes into the picture, 'dependence on the product, the hit, the fantasy productions, dependence on a dealer etc.' (Deleuze, 2007: 153). It is not however discussed who is in the position to decide a drug user's state of dependence and what implications this categorisation has for a drug user's life. Deleuze and Guattari also talk about 'hard' drugs, a classification associated with a moralising system of thought. Overall, the terminology deployed by the two philosophers to talk about drugs is problematic and outdated. The connection between Deleuze and Guattari, and drugs is difficult and troublesome. The content however of their writings, their way of thinking, as well as Deleuze's methodological suggestions in his text *Two Questions on Drugs* (in *Two Regimes of Madness*, 2007) have still a lot to offer.

In *A Thousand Plateaus* (2004), Deleuze and Guattari talk about the drug assemblage as a matter of speed and its modifications, leading to the elimination of forms and persons. For them, the problem with the drug assemblage's line of flight is that it is

> *constantly being segmentarized under the most rigid of forms, that of dependency, the hit and the dose, the dealer ... Instead of making a body without organs sufficiently rich or full for the passage of intensities, drug addicts erect a vitrified or emptied body.*
>
> (Deleuze and Guattari, 2004: 314)

So 'what good does it do to perceive as fast as a quick-flying bird if speed and movement continue to escape somewhere else?' (Deleuze and Guattari, 2004: 314) they ask.

The views of Deleuze and Guattari on dependent drug use are sidelined by empirical researchers who have deployed their theories to talk about the drug assemblage as a dynamic formation. Peta Malins (2004) has provided a critique of what she sees as a deterministic analysis of the drug assemblage. Malins argues that what is problematic about Deleuze and Guattari's analysis is that they put the substance in the centre of the drug assemblage; they focus on the physical effect of the drug and dismiss its aesthetic, spatial, contextual and historical elements. According to Oksanen, Deleuze and Guattari's views on drugs can be attributed to the historical momentum in which they were writing:

> *Deleuze and Guattari were well aware that their attitudes might be interpreted as a positive statement about drugs. When Mille Plateaux was published in 1980, most of the failures of the counterculture and the hippie generation had already been discussed. Deleuze and Guattari wanted to make sure that their ideas of becoming would not be misinterpreted or used as tools in such drug-crazed discourses.*
>
> (Oksanen, 2013: 59)

A close examination of Deleuze's text *Two Questions on Drugs* (2007) might be able to offer a closer insight into the reasons why Deleuze and Guattari understood drug use as a destructive rather than an enabling force. Deleuze does not see all types of drug use under the same prism. He argues that drug use

> *is not suicidal as long as the destructive flow is not reduced to itself but serves to conjugate other flows, whatever the danger. The suicidal enterprise occurs when everything is reduced to this flow alone: 'my' hit, 'my' trip, 'my' glass. It is the contrary of connection; it is organized disconnection.*
>
> (Deleuze, 2007: 154)

Unlike Malins's argument, Deleuze in this account does not focus on the substance itself, or on the act of drug use, but on the individualistic and isolating element of *the way* drugs are used in certain settings and the disconnection from other bodies taking place through the *drug use process.* According to Deleuze, the drug assemblage *does* transform the body, but it does so in an isolating, disempowering way.

Guattari, in his own writings, is equally sceptical towards regular drug use that he sees as another expression of microfascism, a concept that he and Deleuze develop in *A Thousand Plateaus* to answer to the global question why desire desires its own repression (2004: 237):

> *The common characteristic of hard drugs ... appears to me to be the existence of a kind of subjective 'black hole', which I would characterize as microfascist. These black holes continue to multiply, proliferating in the social field. It is a question of knowing if subjectivity echoes them in such a way that the entire life of an individual, all his [sic] modes of semiotization, depend upon a central point of anguish and guilt. I propose this image of a black hole to illustrate the phenomenon of the complete inhibition of the semiotic constituents of an individual or group, which then finds itself cut off from any possibility of an exterior life.*
>
> (Guattari, 1984: 201)

Keane (2002: 34) is also critical of Deleuze and Guattari's description of the drugged body. She argues that although they are not providing a moral or medical judgement but an ethological description of an arrangement of forces, the understanding of the addicted body as frozen and linked could as well describe the recovering addict body, stuck in repetition of a singular truth. She therefore suggests a distinction between Deleuze and Guattari's use of the drugged body as destratified, and the attempts that deploy the writers' vision of corporeality to refigure drug use and addiction (ibid.). Keane's methodological proposal is to shift the question from the good or bad substance to the good or bad encounter:

> *An encounter between a body and a drug could be either a bad poison-like or a good food-like encounter, depending on the specific body, the specific drug*

and the specific situation. The challenge is to increase the good encounters and limit the bad, just as we do in other relationships.

(Keane, 2002: 35)

Keane's proposition to consider and question whether the addicted body's power of acting is interrupted or enhanced while in recovery is an important one. It resonates with the intention to go against generalising statements classifying recovery as 'good' or 'bad', and to focus instead on the encounters becoming within two specific recovery assemblages. A point that needs to be made on Deleuze and Guattari's writings on drugs and the subsequent deployment of their vision of corporeality as a way to talk about drugs is the fact that harm reduction was not yet in the picture. Deleuze and Guattari do not dismiss experimentation with drugs altogether. On the contrary, experimentation is what they primarily focus on (Boothroyd, 2006), potentially not taking into consideration the complexity of other drug realities. They are, for example, very much interested in Antonin Artaud's experimentation with peyote and Henri Michaux's use of mescaline, and although they do not explicitly discuss the relationship between drugs and pleasure, desire and the lines of flight that become possible through drugs are being considered. It is the production and breaking of connections explored in these texts that instigate Deleuze and Guattari's thinking with drugs, as, for example, in the following excerpt, where Artaud accounts for his experimentations with peyote:

The physical hold was still there. This cataclysm which was my body ... After twenty-eight days of waiting, I had not yet come back into myself or, I should say gone out into myself. Into myself, into this dislocated assemblage, this piece of damaged geology ... Twenty-eight days of this heavy captivity, this ill-assembled heap of organs which I was and which I had the impression of witnessing like a vast landscape of ice on the point of breaking up ... And all this, for what? For a dance, for a rite of lost Indians who no longer even know who they are or where they come from and who, when you question them, answer with tales whose connection and secret they have lost.

(Artaud, 1976: 45–46)

Deleuze and Guattari's writings on drugs attempt to account for these questions that remained unanswered by writers and poets that they so much admired. In that sense, their texts on drugs are driven by a certain amount of sentimentality, as they also constitute attempts to make sense of the loss of these people through their encounters with drugs.

In the chapter 'Becoming a drug user – becoming a service-user', I argue that going beyond this explicit deficit of his analysis and some of the terminology deployed, and focusing instead on how Deleuze talks about the connections and encounters that are enabled or blocked through drugs, opens up a line of thought that links his analysis with drug using experiences and renders it empirically relevant. I will specifically discuss, through the accounts of service-users, the methodological suggestions Deleuze makes in *Two Questions on Drugs* (2007), focusing on how causality, turning points and desire can inform our reading of service-users' first experiences with substances.

Overall, by following McLeod and Duff in their Deleuzian methodological approaches, as well as through the empirical deployment of a Deleuzo–Guattarian terminology for the analysis of the service-users' lived experiences of drug use and recovery, my aim is to demonstrate in practice how our reading of recovery as an assemblage can position the desire for care in the focus of attention. Following and accounting for caring practices, as these emerge organically within specific material, affective and social recovery assemblages, can challenge dominant systems that classify recovery engagements as 'failures' or 'successes', ignoring the complexities of people's lives that render these categorisations impossible.

Notes

1 Oksanen has deployed Deleuzian theory to analyse addiction as a situational and interactional process that enables the production of desire. Accordingly, recovery, as he argues, has to activate different possibilities and ensure an open future, produce 'situations and assemblages that modify the everyday interactions between people and things' (2013: 64). This connection between drug treatment and desire is discussed later on in the analysis of the empirical findings. In terms of methodology though, Oksanen has not further explored the specificities of the recovery assemblage. In his ethnographic account, Zigon (2011) also deploys the Deleuzo–Guattarian assemblage to talk about rehabilitation as a space constituted by peculiar global and historical influences. This line of thought though is not further developed, and he only discusses it in relation to the moralities and ethics at play within the rehabilitation programme.

2 In *Anti-Oedipus* (1977), Deleuze and Guattari use the concept 'desiring machine'. The 'assemblage' is the evolution of this concept and first appears in *A Thousand Plateaus* (2004) (Oksanen, 2013: 60).

Chapter 3

Methods as connection-building devices

The theoretical and empirical focus of this book is on connections and care. Within a feminist standpoint, relating and caring are inextricable. 'Relations of thinking and knowing require care', and accordingly 'to care about something, or for somebody, is inevitably to create relation' (de la Bellacasa, 2012: 198). From a Deleuzo–Guattarian perspective, the process of establishing relations between heterogeneous parts (DeLanda, 2016: 2), brings and holds an assemblage together. In the research process, methods are the components mobilised for the production of connections between the researcher and the specific sites and subjects of her research. In other words, they are *connection-building devices* that situate the researcher and the knowledge that a project produces within the specific sites where empirical research takes place. The choice of methods entails the location of the researcher in the field. This 'field' is not stable; a solid terrain where one just enters. Furthermore, the possibilities of the knowledge produced through the encounter of the researcher with the field are not known in advance. When the intention is to leave space for participants to transform research in unexpected ways a commitment to 'mobile positioning' (Haraway, 1988: 585) is required.

My choice of fieldsites was influenced by my working experience in recovery services in Greece and the UK. In Athens, I collaborated with the drug recovery centre 18 ano, an organisation I had worked with in the past, while I was training in art therapy. Through my previous involvement with the service I had already established a relationship of trust with members of staff, and I was familiar with the recovery approach of the programme. In Liverpool I collaborated with Genie in the Gutter, a drug and alcohol, recovery focused, day centre. Unlike 18 ano, I was not familiar with their work in advance, so I offered to volunteer for the service before asking service-users to participate in the study. The willingness to become part of the 'team' while conducting research, rather than to take the role of an external observer, was essential for the establishment of trust relationships with workers and service-users.

While volunteering for the collaborating services and getting to know the service-users, I started conducting interviews with members of staff, including

DOI: 10.4324/9781003165613-4

a wide range of professionals from different backgrounds, holding various positions and responsibilities within the services. At 18 ano I interviewed 13 workers in total: four psychotherapists, five art therapists, one social worker, one volunteer, the head of the research and education department and the manager of one of the social-reintegration guest houses. At Genie I interviewed all permanent members of staff (the CEO and co-founder, the project manager, the project co-ordinator and the key worker) as well as one volunteer. I also conducted interviews with two people that have worked in various drug and alcohol services in the area of Merseyside and one social worker who has working experience in the field of drug use and recovery in both Greece and the UK. For both fieldsites, the main subjects discussed through the interviews were changes in the profiles of service-users, the involvement of the state in the delivery of recovery through the design of drug policies, the needs of the drug using population and how recovery services respond to them, and the difficulties drug and alcohol workers face in the everyday practice of their responsibilities. Additionally, and depending on the specific experience and role of each member of staff, more issues were discussed, like the role of art therapy in the recovery process, the history of the two services, and the working relationships between members of staff.

Building connections with people in recovery

I volunteered at Genie for approximately four months. My responsibilities included attending the team's handover at the beginning and end of each day, sitting at the reception with service-users, and participating in recovery and other groups. It was agreed that the best way to become familiar with the service-users was to co-facilitate recovery groups with the key worker, and after some time I ran the recovery groups as the main facilitator. Additionally, I was attending various other creative and wellbeing groups with the service-users, including dance therapy, art and design, guitar lessons and yoga.

At 18 ano I worked as a volunteer for five months and my main responsibility was to assist with the facilitation of three weekly art-therapy groups in the residential and social re-integration stage of the programme. In the residential stage I was co-facilitating the art group with an art therapist who had also been my instructor during my training at 18 ano. Through drawing and art history, the aim of the specific group is twofold: to encourage service-users to reflect on the relationships between them, and to present art as an aesthetics that can improve people's everyday lives. In the social reintegration stage, I was attending the theatre group. In this group the service-users, directed by a drama therapist, rehearse and perform each year a different play. During the period of my fieldwork I attended rehearsals and presentations of Euripides's 'Medea' and later on rehearsals for Mike Kane's play 'The boy with the suitcase'. The aim of the plays chosen is to give to service-users the opportunity to reflect on their own lives, feelings and experiences, through their relationships with the characters of the play, as well as to work on their personal exposure and confidence.

My presence in both fieldsites was defined by multiple attributions (recovery worker in the past, sociology researcher in the present and volunteer throughout). Consequently, my position as an 'insider' or 'outsider' was complicated. Although in drug ethnographies these terms are mobilised to describe where the researcher stands in relation to the everyday lives and practices of her participants (Maher, 1997; Moore and Measham, 2006), in my case I had to consider whether I stand 'inside' or 'outside' the services I was collaborating with, and how this decision would affect my relationship with service-users. My choice was to stand 'inside' each service and act as a member of staff. I cannot know how this choice affected my relationship with service-users. It might have stopped them from sharing some experiences with me or it might have increased their trust in my intentions. However, considering the experiences of other researchers, the chances are that having already gained the approval of the collaborating services and my acceptance as a volunteer, made the likelihood of resistance to my presence low (Knight, 2015).

Throughout my fieldwork I was standing 'in-between' in various different ways. To start with I was standing in-between two services, in different contexts and with different treatment approaches, attempting to make sense of the connections bringing them closer. Secondly, I was in-between the academia and the recovery workers, as a researcher whose approach is informed by her previous experience as a worker in the field. Additionally, I was standing in-between full-time members of staff and service-users, as a volunteer who is expected to follow rules and boundaries but does not share the same responsibilities as permanent members of staff do. Finally, in relation to the service-users I was in-between the position of a volunteer and a researcher. Although I was performing tasks that volunteers do, I was asking more questions and, through the interviews and the photography projects, I spent more time with them and got to know them in a different way that I would have, if my only identity had been that of a volunteer.

This in-between-ness led to self-reflection in relation to my standpoint that was constantly renegotiated through my multiple attributions in the field. 'In-between-ness' rendered me aware in practice, of how our standpoints affect the situated knowledges we produce (Haraway, 1988) and what it means, when conducting empirical research, to view from a body, rather than to view from above (Strathern, 2004). Occupying my own 'unique' position in the field, revealed the uniqueness and particularity of each service, as well as the uniqueness of the connections created within the services. 'In-between-ness' became an alternate standpoint, both methodologically and empirically.

Emilie Gomart's (2004) empirical research at a drug substitution treatment clinic in France provides an example of how ethical standpoints and awareness of the researcher's positionality produce situated knowledges. Gomart entered the clinic in the hope of finding something *other* than well-rehearsed theories of action (2004: 85, emphasis in original). This *other* became apparent through her presence in the clinic, and her attentiveness to the connections produced between the service workers, the service-users and the substance. What is interesting in her approach is her quest not for participants, but for 'colleagues' amongst all the actors involved:

> *Rather than starting from an identification with drug users, I searched for 'colleagues' among care professionals and drug users who asked the same questions as myself. I would not assume they were like me; but I would allow that others pose questions with me. My aim became to describe the setting in which they asked these questions and the experimentations that they were able to deploy in such settings.*
>
> (Gomart, 2004: 86, emphasis in original)

Overall, when the researcher's access to the field is ensured or enabled by their collaboration with services, issues of positionality need to be addressed. Maher mentions that her 'role as a novice health professional also gave [her] a dimension other than (passive) researcher' (2002: 315), affecting her gaze and analysis of the workers' and participants' practices. Knight (2015), an ethnographer and outreach worker for over a decade, addresses the issue through her acknowledgement that her 'multiple attributions potentially created multiple social positions for [her]' (Knight, 2015: 26). More importantly, these multiple attributions are also reflected in her analysis, where she demonstrates awareness, concern and care, by 'taking seriously' all actors (Knight, 2015: 233). 'Taking seriously' refers to the researcher's commitment to not look for 'blame' among those that deliver or experience recovery, but to follow and unfold the complexities of the recovery process. I have attempted to follow Knight in this respect, and it has not been an un-troubling task. Operating in two different fieldsites where recovery was practised in different ways required a certain element of adaptability of my own understanding and previous experience of how recovery 'should be done'. Committing to the way of operation chosen by each service was the outcome of a process, of building connections with the organisation and service-users, as well as becoming attentive to the connections and practices of care already in place. This positionality derives from my intention to stand with the services, become enthusiastic about their practices, and allow myself to be surprised by them (Gomart, 2004). Therefore, methods are deployed as devices for the creation of stronger connections; ones that derive from the consistent presence of the researcher in the field and can account for her positionality, while embracing the complexity of fieldwork.

My presence as a volunteer and group co-facilitator prior to asking people for interviews was essential for what Stengers refers to as the production of rapport, without which there is no production of knowledge (Stengers,

2011: 62 cited in Vitellone, 2018). Thinking with Stengers, the aim of my presence in the recovery centres in Liverpool and Athens was not simply to become familiar with service-users and so get their permission to record their stories, but mainly to create this rapport that would constitute them as allies in the research process rather than objects of research.

Building connections through interviewing service-users

Interviewing as a research method produces an encounter between the researcher and the participant that transforms both parties involved. The research encounter is an 'event' where assemblages configure (McLeod, 2017: 28). An event where the 'I' of both the researcher and the researched as static and singular subjects is unsettled (Jackson and Mazzei, 2013: 266) and better understood as always becoming (ibid.: 269). In what follows I discuss how I experienced the 'interview event' by focusing on (a) the methods used and the connections made possible through their deployment and (b) the impact of the interview spaces created on the content and emotional framework of the stories told.

At 18 ano I was attending groups as a volunteer at both the residential and the social reintegration stage of the programme. Although I felt my presence in the residential stage was essential for the creation of stronger connections with service-users, all participants were recruited from the final stage of the programme, namely 'social reintegration'. My decision not to recruit participants from the residential stage was based on the fact that it is a time when people work intensively on themselves through one-to-one psychotherapy, group psychotherapy and various art therapy groups. This process can cause emotional vulnerability and asking people to reflect on their first experiences of drug use at that point could have been stressful and potentially impact negatively on their therapeutic process.

In Athens, I interviewed in total 15 service-users, 6 women and 9 men, from the ages of 25 to 45 who had been using drugs for 7 to 35 years. With the exception of one participant whose drug of choice was benzodiazepines, all others reported heroin as the primary substance of use. Apart from heroin being their preferable substance, the majority of the participants considered themselves poly-drug users of various substances including cocaine, sisa,[1] cannabis, benzodiazepines and alcohol.

The recruitment of participants at Genie was done in a similar way. I initially discussed my project in the recovery group, inviting service-users to take part and then printed out information on the research and left some copies at the reception area. At Genie there are no different 'stages' of recovery, and the service does not offer psychotherapy but practical and emotional support around addiction and other related issues.

In terms of gender representation, approximately 20% of Genie's service-users identify as female and 80% as male. This gender imbalance derives from the fact that male service-users tended to remain engaged with the service for longer periods of time than female ones. As discussed with members of staff, the inconsistency of female clients could potentially be attributed to the fact that male service-users, except for outnumbering the female ones, also tend to be more vocal in groups, rendering it more difficult for women to claim their own space. This was eventually addressed by Genie through the establishment of a weekly women's only group.

In total I interviewed 11 Genie service-users, 8 men and 3 women, from the ages of 31 to 71 who had been using substances for 2 to 49 years. For most of them the substances of choice were alcohol, cocaine and cannabis. Only two participants named heroin and other opioids as their drug of choice. Apart from the participants identifying as alcoholics (6), the others reported poly-drug use.

Becker's methods and space-specific stories of drug use and recovery

For the interview structure I followed Howard Becker's approach in *Becoming a Marihuana User* (1953), in order to trace participants' drug use from the time the use of substances became 'possible and desirable' (Becker, 1953: 235) to the time they started identifying their use as problematic. The main pre-rogative was the exploration of the shifting desire from learning to be a drug user to learning to be a service-user, and the emergence of the recovering subject through this process. Going beyond the identification of facts, traits and causes, the emphasis was on the participants' descriptions of the set of changes in their conception of drug use and of the experiences it provided them (Becker, 1953: 235).

Through discussions on the components – people, objects, places, feelings – that formed a person's first encounter with the drug assemblage, a mapping of the substance's territory came into being. Talking about the initial positive affect of substance use, opened up an analysis of how desire invested and gradually shaped the body's system of perception. The map coming into being throughout the interviews was not static but fluid, as discussions moved on from early experiences of drug use to the substances becoming fundamental components of the participants' subjectivities. The identification of drug use as problematic was then explored through the set of environmental, social and emotional 'changes in the person's conception of the activity' (Becker, 1953: 235).

Becker's study *Becoming a Marihuana User* was published in 1953, and remains present in the methodological and epistemological debates on the problem of description in the social sciences (Vitellone, 2021). It constitutes one of the first attempts to reject the (common at the time) comprehension of the drug user as a pathological subject, and to focus instead on social practices that render drug use possible and desirable. Through the methodological deployment of the Deleuzo–Guattarian assemblage for the unpacking of the complexity of the recovery process, I have taken Becker's approach one step further. Following the history of the participants' relationship with substances, I invited them to complicate their stories by sharing how drug use can become simultaneously possible and impossible, desirable and painful, and how their drug experiences came to be renegotiated through the recovery experience.

Following marihuana users' shifts from 'unexperienced' to 'experienced' users, Becker empirically demonstrated that 'between trying it [marihuana] for the first time and being a regular user, there is a necessary learning process' (Pessin, 2017: 15). What the novice user has to *learn* if they want to follow a drug using career is how to experience drug use as a desirable and pleasurable activity. According to Becker this is a social process, as the knowledge does not directly derive from the relationship between the substance and the user, but from active participation in the environments where drug use happens. A close observation of how 'experienced' users relate to the drug, how they hold it and smoke it, as well as how they experience being 'high', is the way to experience drug use in a similarly pleasurable way. Working however with people who have voluntarily engaged with recovery services, demonstrates that 'learning' how to be a user does not permanently ensure pleasurable drug experiences. Therefore, instead of asking participants about the learning process that rendered substance use pleasurable, I was more interested in the assemblages that rendered substance use desirable. By following, through their narratives, the interruptions of the flows of desire, initially enabled through the encounter with the substance, I moved on to ask them about the emergence of another desire, the desire to *learn how to become a recovering subject*. The drug assemblage (where one learns how to become a user) is thus discussed through the interviews in parallel with the recovery assemblage (where one learns how to become a service-user), mirroring each other and exploring the associations and connections between the production of the drug using space and the production of the recovery space.

Building connections through the interview event

Stories are not told in isolation but become with the spaces, bodies and affects, as these come together for the production of contexts (Duff, 2014a; Sultan and Duff, 2021). Although experiences of substance use were extensively discussed during the interviews, it is important to emphasise that these are *space-specific recovery stories*, in the sense that they were produced at a time when both the participants and the researcher were part of the recovery assemblage. The connections created between us were enhanced and mediated by the affective flows that hold the assemblage together. The specific differences in the approach and practice of recovery in the two collaborating services will be discussed in the next chapter. I here reflect (a) on how the approaches of the services affect the narratives of their service-users, positioning the interview event *within, and as part of the recovery assemblage* and (b) on how the interactions between the researcher and the participants potentially shaped the stories told. I therefore account for the connections enabled through interviews, as these emerged within two different recovery assemblages.

The state in which the interviewer and the interviewee enter the interview event is an encounter between subjectivities that carry with them certain experiences and expectations. It is not only the interviewee's cognitively articulated sense of self that is co-created by both parties, through the questions asked, but also the emotional framing of the story that is co-shaped by the emotional stances of the interviewer and the interviewee (Ezzy, 2010: 168). Maher describes the relationship between the ethnographer and her informant(s) as one where 'each party draws on her own historical experiences to make sense of "the other"' (Maher, 1997: 231).

Interviews with 18 ano's participants took place *outside* of their structured recovery daily programme. As attendance to psychotherapeutic and art groups taking place at various locations in the city is compulsory for service-users, we had to plan the interviews at times that did not coincide with any therapeutic activities. This meant that both the interviewer and interviewee had to make a specific commitment for the interview to become possible. Although I would always make the effort to arrange interviews at times and places primarily convenient for interviewees, the time spent for the interview was part of their *personal* rather than their *recovery time*. The space thus created for the interview event was somewhere in-between the recovery and the personal space, leading to the production of connections different to the ones service-users and myself had built through structured recovery activities. Although similar boundaries applied in regards to interpersonal relationships, and our meetings were taking place within the premises of the organisation, the themes discussed during the interview were deeper and more personal than the subjects usually addressed in art groups, happening though in a more informal and less structured form than a psychotherapy session would. However, the fact that talking therapy was a big part of 18 ano's participants' lives at the time, rendered them more prepared to share and reflect upon significant and emotional life experiences.

The connections created with service-users of Genie and by consequence the stories told through the interviews, differed significantly from the ones built with the service-users of 18 ano. Genie is a day centre with specific opening days and times. The service-users are welcome to spend the whole day there (9am–5pm) even if they are not willing to attend all activities taking place throughout the day. As a result, my interviews with participants were scheduled to take place on week days between 9am and 5pm, *within* the recovery space and time. In that sense, the commitment required from their part – in terms of the structure of their day, not in relation to their emotional commitment to the project – was not additional, but part of their commitment to attend the service at a specific day. Therefore, unlike my experience at 18 ano where the interview space created, shifted the nature of my connection with the participants, at Genie the interview space would be better described as an extension of the recovery space. Overall, the content as well as the emotional framework of the stories told in both fieldsites was affected by similar components, leading not only to the production of different stories between the two fieldsites, but also to the creation of different connections. While with the participants of 18 ano, my presence in the recovery assemblage marked the beginning of a connection-building process that was strengthened through the interviews, my connection with Genie's service-users was created and negotiated within the recovery groups, with the interviews being an expression of established trust.

Finally, it was also gender realities, roles and experiences affecting the connections created between the researcher and the service-users. My interview interactions with female participants of 18 ano are indicative of the ways in which gender affects the spaces created for interviews, and by extension the stories told. At 18 ano when I first asked people to participate, with just one exception, it was only men that signed up. Men were more eager to talk and trust me with their experiences; the process of building trust relationships with women took longer. However, once such a relationship had been established, women were more likely to share their personal and occasionally sensitive and traumatic experiences of drug use. This was mainly observed in relation to stories of physical and sexual abuse. Although this was not a subject explicitly questioned during the interviews, for female participants the narration of their lives as drug users was usually accompanied by such an incident. While experiences of abuse are also common for male drug users (Liebschutz et al., 2002; Schneider et al., 2008), male participants hardly ever described in detail cases of abuse, potentially due to gender norms around disclosure of sexual victimisation (Javaid, 2015; Turchik and Edwards, 2012).

Building connections through photography

In qualitative research on drug use, visual methods and especially photography-based research methods have been deployed in various different ways, primarily as a means to position in the centre of attention the everyday realities of drug users (Bourgois and Schonberg, 2009; Fitzgerald, 2002; Knight, 2015).

My way of working with photography with participants reflects McLeod's (2017) use of photography with people with depression. McLeod deploys photography as a way to make materials central and active, and to direct her attention to non-human action. Her participants planned, took, and edited their photos in their own time, and then delivered 'a rehearsed narrative about each photo' (McLeod, 2017: 31) through one to one encounters, where 'the photos were the key communicative device ... The position [that McLeod] moved to in these encounters was simply to be present and witness the affective force or sensation of the photos' (ibid.: 33). In turn, my encounters with the participants were driven by the photographs and the photographers' narratives. My involvement was limited to asking for some clarifications, rather than having a plan in advance about where the discussion was going to go.

Although visual methods remain far from standardised and researchers have defined and used them in various ways (Padgett et al., 2013: 1436), the way photography was deployed in this project is closer to what has been defined as photovoice. 'Photovoice has emerged from the fields of health and community assessment studies as a photo elicitation technique that facilitates participant involvement at all stages of the research process' (Given et al., 2011). According to Harper, 'photo elicitation is based on the simple idea of inserting a photograph into a research interview' (Harper, 2002: 13). What photovoice adds to this idea is the requirement that the images used in the interviews should be participant generated. I chose the specific method for two main reasons, with the first one being to empower participants to engage more deeply in the research process by being in control of how the images are used (Given et al., 2012). Secondly, the process of taking photographs as well as their subsequent discussion, provided a closure to the issues explored during the interviews, whose aim was to record the drug using and recovering stories of participants in specific spaces and times. Elicitation interviews open up an opportunity for the connection of '"core definitions of the self" to society, culture and history' (Harper, 2002: 13), and offer an 'approach that takes seriously participants as knowers' (Guillemin and Drew, 2010: 177). Asking participants to re-visit their chosen spaces in the cities where they had experienced drug use and recovery, and to see them through the lens of the camera, created a new connection between them and the spaces they inhabit. Through the discussions on the photographs taken, the aim was to trace the shifting experience of the city as a space of substance use to a space of recovery.

In both Liverpool and Athens, the recruitment process for the photography project was done in parallel with the interviews. At the end of each interview I asked participants whether they would be interested in participating in a photography project, going beyond substance use and exploring how they positioned themselves in the public and private environments they inhabited. From that point onwards, the project followed quite different paths in Athens and in Liverpool.

In Athens, I called a first meeting for the service-users interested in participating in the photography project, with the aim to establish a concrete research subject as well as a way of collaboration. Some of the issues discussed and negotiated during the meeting were whether the focus should be on recovery, personal or public spaces – and it was agreed to focus on public spaces; whether the photographs should be taken individually or within a group – it was agreed to do photography walks as a group; and whether the aim was to depict the past, future or present – it was decided that this would be up to each participant, as long as explicit captures of drug use were avoided. Agreeing on a specific theme in advance was not easy, but the general idea was to focus on the photographic capture of the fears, hopes and concerns that people in recovery deal with when trying to re-integrate as equal members in the social environments they inhabit. By re-visiting a given urban space through photography, our aim was to address the city as a complex apparatus where personal stories, memories and desires coexist and are shaped in parallel with historical, social and cultural collective narratives.

Following our initial meeting, the group met overall four more times; twice to take photos and twice to discuss them. For our first photography walk we met at the area of Kypseli, currently one of the most ethnically and financially diverse areas of Athens (Maloutas, 2004; Vaiou, 2010). Our second photography walk started at the flea market of Monastiraki, and continued up to Athinas street until Omonoia square. The particularity of this area is that it is simultaneously an attraction for tourists, a shopping area for the locals and a space of drug dealing and use. It was chosen exactly because of these characteristics which are also telling of the urban and social structure of Athens overall (Leontidou, 2012; Noussia and Lyons, 2009).

With the participants from Genie, the photography project was conducted in a different way. Unlike 18 ano, where service-users are already familiar with group work and prepared to share their experiences in such a setting, groups at Genie operate differently. Service-users are asked to refrain from sharing very personal or traumatic experiences as the group dynamic is such that confidentiality cannot be guaranteed. They are encouraged to discuss primarily issues that have to do with their everyday lives, triggers to use or drink, and coping mechanisms they develop. Additionally, the groups do not always have the same structure as service-users can show up at any time and day during the week and attend the activities scheduled. It was therefore decided that participants will take photos individually and at their own time, and the analysis of the photographs took place through one-to-one conversations.

Most of the participants from Genie were using old mobile phones, so in terms of technical support they were provided with one disposable camera each. We agreed in advance that they would keep the cameras for two weeks and then they would return them to me to have the photographs printed. When the photographs were ready, we renewed our appointment to discuss them. Before meeting them, I had scanned the photographs so that after the discussion they could keep the ones I had already printed out. This was a way to acknowledge that they were the participants' property, to increase their engagement and to establish joint ownership of the project. As the conditions were not suitable for a collective definition of a theme for the photography project, the research subject remained the same as it had been developed with participants from 18 ano.

The differences in the visual methods deployed in the two fieldsites, deriving from the specific characteristic of each recovery assemblage, emphasise the impact of methods on the research assemblages produced. While the group analysis of the photographs taken by the participants of 18 ano provided rich data, our structured photography walks left less time and space for participants to explore and take pictures of locations and objects potentially more significant for them individually, than the neighbourhoods chosen collectively by the group. When, for example, one of the participants took the initiative and brought in our discussion pictures from his place of residence at the time, the analysis went much further and opened up the discussion to the relationship between public and private spaces. The participants of Genie on the other hand, had more time to photograph places, public and private, as well as objects important to them. The subsequent analysis of the pictures followed different paths, primarily focused on their memories from the places and objects they had chosen to capture. The different ways of working with photography demonstrate that 'participants are not passive data providers but actors in the research whose choices influence the results and outcomes' (Given et al., 2012). Finally, it shows in practice the ways in which the connections built through methods reflect the particularities of each recovery assemblage.

Building connections between services

The aim of this book is to challenge fixed knowledges, and open up a space for the exploration of the deterritorialisations that become possible within the recovery assemblage. Following this commitment, analysis has been consistent with the methodological deployment of the Deleuzo–Guattarian assemblage, to unfold the flows and practices of care that render possible the transition from the drug using to the recovering subject. The voices of participants are not discussed as factual and individual 'truths' but as testimonies of how 'the subject is *produced in thought and practice*' (Duff, 2014a: 28, emphasis in original). The stories narrated through the interviews are not treated as linear accounts of individual lives but as shared experiences of the transformations of the using and the recovering body, when connected with other bodies and with objects and spaces (Duff, 2007: 515).

Staying committed to render visible the connections becoming within, but also *between* different recovery assemblages, I work with the visual and oral data produced *as one body in becoming*. The participants' accounts becoming in the two recovery assemblages are not discussed separately, but brought together through the connections they enable. In practice this means that I have refrained from specifying whether the data discussed were produced in Athens or Liverpool.[2] Stengers distinguishes between measurements 'acting like a unilateral sieve, retaining only what can be measured, and measurements as related to the *creation* of a rapport or *logos*' (Stengers, 2011: 49–50, emphasis in original). Following Stengers, I am not concerned with findings that would derive from measurable qualities and would make a statement about best and worst practices. My interest is in the connections created within each service and in the ones that become possible by thinking about recovery through data produced in two different recovery assemblages. Furthermore, both recovery assemblages of Liverpool and Athens are components of the wider assemblage of recovery (DeLanda, 2016), as it traverses specific spatial and historical boundaries. The relations assembled across the research encounters (McLeod, 2017: 31) go beyond specific territorialities and produce knowledge on the relations and connections becoming possible within the recovery space, and through sociological empirical research overall.

In the next chapter the structural differences between the collaborating services will be addressed, situating them in history and policy. I now want to briefly outline some of the recovery components shared by Genie and 18 ano, practices and approaches that enhance the connections built within each service, and enable the connections between them. These common elements are (1) The emphasis on art and creative activities as part of the recovery process. Art and creative activities within a group setting create connections through a shared manual labour and leave space for the unspoken to be shared; the feelings that cannot be talked about but are communicated through the production of works of art. (2) The confrontational relationship between the services and the state, to be addressed in the next chapter and (3) The inclusion of people with mental health issues alongside their drug use, discussed in the previous chapter. The aim here is twofold: firstly, to understand both services in their uniqueness and particularity, and secondly to explore the connections between these two entities.

Finally, I did not attempt to allocate pseudonyms to the participants and, when quoting them, I do not mention their age, gender or any other characteristic that could lead to assumptions about their identities. In doing so, my intention is to respect their anonymity as much as their actual names and lives. Renaming, whether it is done by the researcher or the participants themselves is not an 'innocent' process. It reflects issues of power and voice, and methodological choices (Allen and Wiles, 2016; Lahman et al., 2015). Disclosing gender and age can also, intentionally or unintentionally, lead to speculations about why one talks in one way or another. Therefore, revealing certain aspects of one's identity but not others would not do justice to the actual lives and identities of the people involved in this research, and furthermore could unwittingly lead to categorisations and classifications.

Both Genie and 18 ano did not only consent to be named, but were actively keen on their recovery practices being widely communicated. The majority of the workers also consented to be named, but I have done so only in cases where it was essential for the flow of the narration. I decided against naming all of them for reasons of consistency – a few of them felt more comfortable in maintaining anonymity – and to avoid confusing the readers with names. However, I have not tried to anonymise them further by refraining for example from stating their job titles.

Throughout the book I refer to the participants as service-users. In 18 ano, those engaging with the service are referred to as 'therapeuomenoi', which literally translates into 'the ones in therapy'. This term reflects the psychotherapeutic approach of the service. In Genie, the people engaging with the service are called 'clients'. Although the word 'clients' implies a financial transaction between the service and its users, it has been widely deployed by free of charge UK drug and alcohol services, like Genie. Both 'therapeuomenoi' and 'clients' are context-specific terms. I have opted for the term 'service-user' instead, as it does not contradict the approach of the collaborating services, and is primarily descriptive, rather than reflective of the services' practices. Throughout the interviews though, as well as in the everyday practices of the services, workers of both Genie and 18 ano referred to service-users through the informal term 'the guys' (for 18 ano that is 'paidia', which literally translates into 'kids', however in Greek it is used in the same way that the word 'guys' is used in English). Overall, the quotes of service-users and workers have not been edited, and I have attempted through the translation of the Greek quotes to maintain the tone of the language used.

The encounter between the researcher and the participant is an event that matters, as it traverses all aspects of empirical studies, from the epistemological and methodological choices made, to the specific methods deployed and the empirical knowledge produced. The chapters that follow are the outcome of these theoretical and methodological choices, as they emerged through my interactions with participants, put into words and analysed through the connections built and the exchanges enabled within the research assemblage.

Notes

1 Sisa is a psychoactive drug from Greece, also known as the 'austerity drug' as it first appeared during the years of the financial crisis and is cheaper than any other illicit drug. Its main ingredient is crystal methamphetamine filled with battery acid or engine oil (Talking Drugs (2012) www.talkingdrugs.org/sisa-the-drug-of-the-poor).

2   There are a few exceptions to this. In cases for example where the discussion is about the specific territoriality of one assemblage or the other, and the public and political spaces within which they evolve, the data produced in Athens and Liverpool are discussed separately. Additionally, in cases where the data discussed are only from one fieldsite, this is mentioned.

Chapter 4

Of other spaces

The birth of the heterotopia of recovery

In his text 'Of other spaces', Foucault argues that in our epoch, space takes for us the form of relations among sites (1986: 23). This is a heterogeneous space that does not come into being inside a void, but through a set of relations that delineates various sites (ibid.: 24). Among these sites, Foucault is interested in the ones that have the 'property of being in relation with all the other sites, but in such a way as to suspect, neutralize, or invent the set of relations that they happen to designate, mirror, or reflect' (ibid.: 25). He names these sites 'heterotopias'. 'Foucault's outlines of heterotopia attempt to explain principles and features of a range of cultural, institutional and discursive spaces that are somehow "different": disturbing, intense, incompatible, contradictory and transforming' (Johnson, 2013: 790). Therefore, heterotopias are not idealised reflections of the societies through which their 'otherness' is established (Hetherington, 1997: 43), but sources of 'ambivalence and uncertainty, thresholds that symbolically mark not only the boundaries of a society but its values and beliefs as well' (ibid.: 49). Accordingly, the time of one's engagement with recovery signifies a break from life as it was before; a rupture with the ways in which life was organised, in order to reflect on it and change it according to new desires that emerge. The heterotopia of recovery becomes in relation to other sites but is different to them; it reflects them, but also attempts to transform them by allowing ambiguity and uncertainty to be expressed. Recovery is a heterotopia of contemplation, embedded in aspects of one's life, mirroring them but also unsettling and inverting them (Johnson, 2013: 790–791). In what follows I address the histories of the recovery spaces I have been collaborating with in Athens and Liverpool, focusing on how these heterotopias came into being.

In the previous chapter it was mentioned that the two first characteristics of the assemblages as these were identified by DeLanda (2016) – their contingent historical identity that constitutes them individual entities, and their composition of heterogeneous components – will be discussed following Foucault's heterotopology. I account for the histories of the recovery assemblages I worked with, as these became through their entanglement with the contexts

DOI: 10.4324/9781003165613-5

within which they emerged. I do so by exploring how the specific material assemblages were produced in relation (through accordance or conflict) to the policymaking systems and the political and social assemblages they are components of, leading to their current identities and practices. Finally, I argue that by talking about the history of the infrastructure and the institution *in relation* to the people that occupy it, we can account for the becoming of the recovery assemblage, and the ways in which care is practised.

Heterotopias 'are spaces in which an alternative social ordering is performed ... stand[ing] in contrast to the taken-for-granted mundane idea of social order that exists within society' (Hetherington, 1997: 40). By positioning the emergence of the recovery assemblage within specific policymaking, social and political contexts, and driven by the lived experiences of service-users, I closely attend to the specificities of the recovery assemblage's alternative ordering, and the alternative connections that this ordering enables, accounting for the ways in 'which [they] rupture the order of things through their different mode of ordering to that which surrounds them' (Hetherington, 1997: 46). Addressing the 'otherness' of the recovery assemblage, the need for the generation of an alternative ordering, complicates the relationship between policymaking and the birth of drug services. The history of the drug services I am exploring has been antagonistic to policymaking practices, where the latter have been often conceived and applied as mechanisms mobilised to interrupt the recovery assemblage's alternative ordering.

Drug use and recovery in Greece: the birth of 18 ano

Treatment of drug use is one area in which European countries have not always followed traditional strategies, although they are all bound to the same treaties,[1] but have developed individual and nationalised approaches (Chatwin, 2007: 497). Greece's modern history of drug use and recovery has always been one step behind the rest of the Western world (Yfantis, 2017; Matsa, 2007), with drug use abruptly appearing in the Greek press as 'a major social issue' in the middle of the 1980s (Tsili, 1995). Another particularity of the Greek case that has affected the recent history of drug use and recovery is the very low rate of HIV positive drug users up until 2012 (Nikolopoulos et al., 2015). The above characteristics of the Greek case need to be taken into consideration, when trying to comprehend the reasons why, while in the rest of Europe attention turned to harm reduction in an attempt to minimise the effects of the so-called HIV crisis, in Greece the focus remained on abstinence-based, residential drug treatment services. Finally, the last element that needs to be introduced is the absence of concrete drug policies and the lack of governmental interventions on the treatment and recovery models applied (Fotopoulou and Parkes, 2017; Kokkevi et al., 2000). Despite the state's punitive approach to drug use and possession, drug policy has never attempted to regulate, change or control the provision of drug treatment

(Tragakes and Polyzos, 1998). Therefore, the main public drug recovery programmes, still active today, had the opportunity to develop their own therapeutic approaches, while maintaining their public funding.

KETHEA (Centre for the Therapy of Addicted Persons), the first semi-public drug treatment centre to appear in Greece, was first established in 1983 with the operation of a detoxification centre and a day centre. Shortly afterwards it opened its first therapeutic community (TC), based on the standards of Emiliehoeve, a famous Dutch TC that had already been the role model for many others operating in Europe around that time (Kooyman, 2001). For many years KETHEA and 18 ano were the only public providers of drug treatment, until the establishment of OKANA (Organisation Against Drugs) in 1996, a publicly funded programme that focuses on methadone maintenance treatment. Up until the establishment of OKANA, the only treatment centre that was created directly by the state, the provision of treatment was not instigated by policymaking practices but by grassroots initiatives that grew to become publicly funded recovery services. Therefore, TCs (KETHEA) and other long-term, residential, abstinence-based programmes (18 ano) prevailed as treatment methods.

Talking about the first principle of heterotopology, Foucault makes a distinction between heterotopias of crisis and heterotopias of deviation. Heterotopias of crisis were privileged or sacred or forbidden places of the so-called primitive societies, 'reserved for individuals who are, in relation to society and to the human environment in which they live, in a state of crisis: adolescents, menstruating women, pregnant women, the elderly, etc.' (1986: 26). In our era the heterotopias of crisis are disappearing and are being replaced by heterotopias of deviation, spaces created for individuals whose behaviour is deviant in relation to the required means or norms, like rest homes, psychiatric hospitals and prisons (ibid.: 27). The recovery space of 18 ano has followed a different route, shifting from a heterotopia of deviation to a heterotopia of crisis, through changes that took place within the recovery space.

The drug recovery centre 18 ano was born as part of, and administratively still belongs to, the Psychiatric Hospital of Attica. Since 1926 (when the first admission of a Greek drug user was registered, see Yfantis, 2017) and up until the 1980s, the common route for drug users and alcoholics was their voluntary or forced admission to the Psychiatric Hospital of Attica (known as Dafni). In 1960, one of the psychiatrists working at Dafni, Rasidakis, established for the first time a system for the classification of the patients. Up until that point, divisions were made based on gender and on whether patients were 'calm' or 'restless'. The classification suggested by Rasidakis was not escaping the psychiatric model, but for the time and within the Greek context, it was the first step towards a different treatment of patients. Following this classification, in 1961, a department specifically for drug users and alcoholics was created within the Psychiatric Hospital of Attica (interview with 18 ano's head of research, January 2018). Within the heterotopic space that the psychiatric hospital is, another heterotopia of deviance was created specifically for drug and alcohol users. In 1972 the department was relocated to the upper floor of the building 18 of the hospital, where the name of 18 ano comes from ('ano' [άνω] in Greek means 'upper'). The recovery principles of the programme, as they still stand today, were set in 1987, when the employees of 18 ano at the time, decided to render treatment voluntary rather than compulsory and stopped accepting mandatory admissions following court orders. This decision marked the transition from a heterotopia of deviance to a heterotopia of crisis, with the difference that what constituted a state of 'crisis' was not defined by the ones responsible for the maintenance of social norms. The decision to 'withdraw' from society into the recovery space had to be made by the person feeling they were in a state of crisis, the drug or alcohol user in need of an 'other' space, different to the sites associated with drug use. Therefore, the primary difference with Foucault's heterotopias of crisis and deviance is that as the recovery space evolved, the authority to identify what constitutes a state of crisis was passed on from the social body to the individual that was experiencing the crisis.

This shifting identity of the recovery space reflects Foucault's second principle of heterotopias: as its history unfolds, an existing heterotopia might function in a very different fashion (1986: 27). In the case of 18 ano, a space of confinement was transformed into a space of treatment, by the people inhabiting it: the workers and service-users of 18 ano at the time. This shift was initiated by the rejection of medicalisation in the treatment of addiction. Within the heavily medicalised space that the psychiatric hospital was, a different space came into being. Drug prescription and substitution were rejected, and psychotherapy and art therapy were deployed as the main treatment methods, setting the foundations of 18 ano as it stands today. As the head of research of 18 ano recalls:

> some of the nurses … left. They left because when they were told that they will have to take the white shirt off and on top of that they have to attend seminars and that we won't be giving meds like we used to and they will have to hang out with the guys [service-users] while they're there, all this didn't go down well because they were like: I'm a nurse, what's all this?

In other words, this shift from a medicalised to a social, psychotherapeutic and anthropocentric approach simultaneously signified a shift of the care provided. While in the past, the primary responsibility of staff was the administration of medicines, in the 'new' 18 ano, they had to take the white shirt off, to symbolically and practically reject their differentiation from the service-users based on their medical expertise. Additionally, they had to hang out with the service-users, to be present for them not as doctors or nurses, but as allies in a recovery process denuded from its past hierarchical mode of operation. This transition of care was also reflected on the organisation of the territoriality of the recovery space. It was at that same period that 18 ano was transformed from an area of confinement to an open house:

> *There were bars everywhere. You would go up the stairs where the office of the nurses was and then another door with bars going into a massive vestibule with high ceilings and then four doors for the four wards, where there were bars too ... At some point it was decided that we can't operate like that anymore, we're not a psychiatric clinic so we don't need the bars so we cut them all down ... and of course the door was open because it was well known from the beginning that whoever wanted to leave could just leave ... That's when, symbolically really, the whole thing became obvious, that we're now something different (from the rest of the psychiatric hospital).*
>
> (interview with 18 ano's head of research, January 2018)

This transformation of 18 ano from a heterotopia of deviance to one of crisis was the Greek response to the anti-psychiatric movement, as it was put in action by radical pedagogues and psychiatrists like the brothers Jean and Fernand Oury in France, and Franco Basaglia and Franco Rotelli in Italy. In 1953, Jean Oury founded the psychiatric clinic La Borde and, together with Felix Guattari, who worked there from 1955 until his death in 1992, they set the foundations of institutional psychotherapy, an approach based on the active participation of the patients in the everyday running of the facility (Genosko, 2009). As part of his involvement with institutional psychotherapy, in 1989, Guattari travelled to Greece to report back on the psychiatric hospital of Leros, notorious for its cruel practices and terrible living conditions of its patients. While in Greece, he also visited 'Dafni', equally infamous at the time for its overcrowded clinics and the de-humanisation of its patients. The thoughts and experiences of Guattari from this journey were recorded in the short book *De Leros à La Borde* (2015), where he provides a brief insight to the position that 18 ano was occupying within Dafni at the time:

> *In order to raise my morale, Chiara Strutti[2] explains to me that in another wing the patients are not constrained anymore. And like a Deus ex Machina, or like a happy end, we find ourselves in a model clinic for thirty drug addicts and alcoholics ... the walls have been painted by the personnel and the patients. Here all methods of one-to-one and group therapy are used (music, psycho-drama, relaxation techniques) ... But the clinic is relatively unknown because of its operation within Dafni, that has such a bad reputation.*
>
> (2015: 57–58)

The becoming heterotopia of 18 ano was also drawing its practices from the recovery centre Marmottan, in France. The psychiatrist Claude

Olievenstein, worked for years with drug and alcohol users incarcerated in psychiatric hospitals and identified the need for a separation between drug users and other mental health patients. He argued for the creation of a new, publicly funding and free institution, where treatment would be voluntary and the focus would be on the abolishment of barriers between staff and drug users, and the creation of affective relations (Olievenstein, 1977: 181). In 1971, following negotiations with the government, Olievenstein was offered Marmottan, an old surgery hospital that had been abandoned. According to the recovery model developed in Marmottan, addiction was a new pathology that should not be identified as an illness, mental or physical, but as a psychological and social issue. The treatment approaches offered varied and included a wide range of psychotherapeutic and creative methods, as well as support with practical areas of the service-users' lives. In that sense, flexibility from the part of the workers was required in order to keep up with the drug users' diverse needs. Occasionally psychotherapeutic approaches were preferred to deal with certain issues, while other times the same issue could become the matter of a critical group putting into question the role of caregivers. Some service-users were interested in political engagement, while others were looking for a mystical adventure. Marmottan had to be the base of this constellation, the heart that drives it and the institution that protects it (Olievenstein, 1977: 191). Members of staff of 18 ano travelled to France to train in Marmottan, next to Claude Olievenstein. Caring practices and treatment approaches of Marmottan were then adjusted and applied within the Greek context and the therapeutic setting of 18 ano upon their return.

Therefore, 18 ano as it stands today is the outcome of two shifting heterotopias. One is the psychiatric clinic that institutional psychotherapy aspired to turn into a self-organised institution that would assist its patients to re-integrate as equal members of their communities. The second one is the recovery space that derives from the psychiatric clinic, but eventually defects from it, both symbolically and physically, for the creation of a new heterotopia where the temporary physical and mental distance from the community is not imposed but chosen by the service-users, as a way to address their needs while in crisis. However, the dynamic that has traversed the history of 18 ano, in relation to its dependence on a heavily bureaucratised and slow state mechanism, has informed the controversies and problems that remain present in its current operation. The lack of direct political intervention to the way that drug treatment is provided in Greece does not automatically signify the absence of any sort of regulation coming from the state. With the Ministry of Health being either the main or the only source of funding, public recovery programmes are administratively dependent on the state and constantly under the threat of financial drought. It is thus through bureaucratic mechanisms and administrative processes that the control of drug services is achieved. The intervention of the Greek state in the way that drug recovery is delivered has been and is still done by reducing the flexibility of the heterotopia of recovery through its bureaucratisation.

It was earlier argued that the shift of 18 ano from a heterotopia of confinement to one that remains penetrable was symbolically achieved through the rejection of medicalisation, and through the service's differentiation from the psychiatric clinic within which it belonged. This differentiation was not only accomplished through the caring practices provided, but also through a shift of the ways in which the service was organised. Challenging the psychiatric institution's classification of patients, 18 ano rejected all forms of record keeping about the people engaging with the service, as this was regarded as a medically centred practice. According to 18 ano's head of research:

> *After the bars were cut, 18 ano started living its adolescence, so it started abolishing anything that reminded of a psychiatric clinic. It started with the bars of course so within this logic we also stopped keeping records. The records remind of doctors and we are not medically-centred so we abolished the records. What did we replace them with? Nothing [laughing]. So there was no evidence [about the service-users]. We reached a point that they were asking us from the Ministry [of Health] how many are the service-users and we couldn't tell … In any case, as of 2009 we started using a questionnaire [completed by the service-users] so that we can provide evidence when the administrations asks for it.*

Although eventually this rejection of any record-keeping mechanisms created practical issues, at the time, this refusal to classify service-users as medical subjects, symbolically marked the differentiation of the heterotopia of recovery from the heterotopia of the psychiatric institution. In practice though, 18 ano remained, and still is part of the Psychiatric clinic of Attica, meaning that it is not only dependent on a medical apparatus, but on an administrative one as well. The programme does not have its own budget which means that every request, even for small amounts – like money to buy some tools for gardening – has to be approved by the administration of the Hospital and then by the Ministry of Health. Once the funds are released, they are first given to the hospital and then the administration of the hospital has to give them to the programme. Thus, besides the rejection of medicalisation in theory and practice, paradoxically 18 ano remains fully dependent on a political and medical apparatus. This constant financial and bureaucratic struggle has accompanied its history from the early years until today. As 18 ano's head of research recalls:

> *It was during the heat wave of 1989 and they [service-users] wanted to go to the beach, and we needed 1000[3] drachmas for the petrol and 1000 drachmas for the driver that would take them there and it was impossible to find the*

money. It wasn't that much money but the bureaucracy of the hospital just
wouldn't [approve it], and of course there were no air-conditions.

Although the financial situation of the hospital and accordingly of 18 ano has
not always been that restrictive, the service has always been dependent on the
hospital's bureaucratic mechanisms and, especially after the financial crisis of
2008, it was not only the release of funds for additional activities, but also the
coverage of the service-users' basic needs that became again a difficult task
(Ifanti et al., 2013; Kentikelenis et al., 2014; Kenitkelenis and Papanicolas,
2011). To address these difficulties, for many years now, 18 ano has been
asking for administrative independence from the hospital, while maintaining
its public funding as part of the national health system. This claim has not
been heard by any of the governments from the 1980s until today, with the
only other option being the removal of the service from the national health
system and its establishment as an NGO. This control of treatment services
by the state, through their entanglement with bureaucracy and administrative mechanisms, was recently reflected on the current government's overnight
decision to cease the autonomy of KETHEA, the largest semi-public provider
of treatment services, by replacing its elected, voluntary management board
with a new board of managers from the public and private sector. This action
was regarded by the community of KETHEA, as well as by other recovery
services standing in solidarity with it, as a direct political intervention at the
operation of the service.[4]

Overall, the inability or unwillingness of the Greek governments of the past
30 years to come up with a concrete drug treatment policy has allowed for
the public recovery services to develop their drug treatment approaches in a
bottom-up fashion, free from external interventions. Heterotopias of recovery
thus emerged as spaces where alternative orderings became possible, different
to the societies that surround them. At the same time though, governmental
control has taken other forms, with the main one being the entanglement of
services with bureaucratic and administrative apparatuses, diminishing the
recovery services' flexibility and autonomy, primarily by complicating their
financial streams. This renders the heterotopic space of recovery dependent
on the state, autonomous in its daily mode of operation and yet attached to
mechanisms that guarantee the state's access at any given time.

Drug use and recovery in the UK: the birth of Genie in the Gutter

While in both Greece and the UK the becoming of the recovery assemblages
has been controlled through the provision of funding, in the UK the allocation of funding has been associated with governmental drug-policy strategies that have a direct impact on the provision of drug treatment. This is
quite paradoxical, considering that most drug and alcohol services did not

grow through, and never became part of a state-run institution. They evolved organically, responding to needs that were not being addressed by the national health system, eventually funded by the state but always as external to its formations, usually registered as charities (Mold and Berridge, 2007; Strang and Gossup, 1994). The vulnerability of the 'other spaces' of recovery in the UK is discussed following the history of drug use, services and policies.

UK has its own history of radical (anti)-psychiatric initiatives, with the main one being the 'democratic therapy' model, a significant movement 'for the reform of mental health services, which brought together mental health patients, radical health workers and social and political activists' (Rawlings and Yates, 2001: 14). This new approach was initially applied in the 'democratic treatment communities' that appeared for the first time in England during World War II and were set up to support soldiers who had suffered mental breakdown (Kooyman, 2001). They gradually expanded to include various psychiatric clinics that adopted a horizontal structure where the residents were not treated as patients but as individuals capable of making their own decisions and being equal members of the community. However, unlike the case of 18 ano, the development of drug and alcohol services in the UK has not been associated with national or international radical psychiatric movements. This could be attributed to the fact that drug use was not originally identified as a mental illness, leading to the voluntary or involuntary confinement in psychiatric hospitals, but as a physical one, rendering doctors working in the community the 'experts' originally allocated to address the needs of the drug and alcohol using population. Accordingly, drug services did not emerge through the transformation of existing heterotopias of deviance, but from the increasing need to create 'other' spaces able to provide support going beyond the physical issues associated with regular drug use.

The first UK drug policy document was the 1920s Dangerous Drugs Act,[5] describing drug use as the manifestation of a disease requiring a medical response, and opening the way for the legitimisation of drug prescriptions and substitutes for users. Known as the 'Rolleston report', the document marked a compromise between the US-driven call for a penal approach, and the incorporation of medical professionals in drug treatment (Berridge, 1980), leading to the establishment of the 'British system' (Mars, 2003). Drug users were not 'expelled' from the community to the heterotopia of the psychiatric hospital, to be disciplined by psychiatrists, but treated by doctors within the community through the prescription of substitutes that would render them functional and manageable (Stimson, 1983: 120). The control of doctors over the addicted body was further stressed out in the subsequent drug policy documents of the 1960s[6] through the re-enforcement of the medical model,

by arguing that addiction should be seen as a 'socially infectious' condition. In consequence, the task of the doctors was not only therapy but additionally control of the spread of the disease by controlling the addict and the supply of drugs.

(Stimson, 1983: 120)

Although medical prescriptions and opioid substitutes were the prevailing approach to drug use, TCs for drug and alcohol also grew to occupy a place in the early history of drug and alcohol treatment in the UK. Influenced by the concept-based 'Synanon' in the United States, by the end of the 1960s there were similar, service-users' led TCs, providing an alternative to the medically led substitution-based treatment (for more information on the TC and their UK history see Broekaert, 2001; Kooyman, 2001; Raimo, 2001). These recovery spaces have a lot of similarities with the heterotopias of recovery, appearing at the same time in European countries, but constitute only a small part of UK treatment services, privately funded and sidelined by dominant drug policy discourses.

The type of services leading to the context within which Genie was established, are the ones initially responding to un-met needs of the drug using population. These services later gained governmental funding, in exchange for their adaptation to the demands of official drug policies. I understand these spaces as small heterotopias appearing and disappearing within urban environments, continually struggling between the application of innovative recovery visions and the bureaucratisation and professionalisation necessary for their financial survival. The first example of such a drug service was *Lifeline*, established in Manchester in 1971 by the psychiatrist Dr Eugenie Cheesmond. Lifeline was initially a day centre, offering food to drug users, with the aspiration to become a non-residential TC. Rowdy Yates (1992), a former drug user who later on became the CEO of the organisation, in his account of the history of the project, describes the mistakes, obsessions and disillusionments the Lifeline team went through, while improvising in its attempts to meet the drug users' needs.

Lifeline in its early days was defined by (a) its political characteristics, as it viewed itself to be 'outside the establishment, creating an alternative and better society' (Yates, 1992: 9), (b) its opposition to medicalisation and substitution as 'society had been hypnotised by doctors and drug companies into accepting a chemical intervention for every unpleasant situation' (ibid.) and (c) its dependence on the energy and vision of one charismatic person, Dr Cheesmond, who was setting the rules and was responsible for management. The Lifeline workers of the time, lacking any official and structured training, were developing their skills in practice, while dealing with overdoses and violent conflicts in the day centre. As has been the case with 18 ano and as will be discussed shortly, with Genie too, the locomotive that kept Lifeline going during its first years of operation was enthusiasm. An enthusiasm deriving from the workers' appetite to learn and fight for the provision of care to drug users, as they understood it at the time. Lifeline's informal mode of operation had to be revised when the organisation was given the opportunity to get stable governmental funding. The increase of heroin use at the end of the 1970s (James, 1971; Mitcheson et al., 1970) was faced by the government through the provision of funding to voluntary organisations already in operation (Mold, 2004). This opportunity for financial security of services that had been struggling to make ends meet would not come without a cost:

> *Lifeline Project entered a period of bureaucracy which would have been inconceivable at its inception … Gradually, management became a thing that actually happened, rather than just something we told the funders we did … For the first time since the establishment of England's therapeutic communities in the sixties, there was a bridgehead between the National Health Service and the voluntary sector drugs field … But how did we get there? We hid our outlaw masks and signed on as deputies in a new posse … We thought that we could sort out the ideology later.*
>
> (Yates, 1992: 42–44)

Genie, in relation to its aims and mode of operation, reflects the aspirations of these first drug services. The service was founded by Carolyn Edwards and her brother, who had been through recovery himself.[7] Its name comes from Carolyn's brother's imaginary friend called Genie, an unfinished book that would have been entitled Genie in the Gutter, and an Oscar Wilde quote 'we're all in the gutter but some of us look at the stars'. It was born in 2008, responding to the lack of services at the time able to provide a holistic support to people taking their first steps in the recovery process, but were not ready to maintain abstinence. It was the organisation of a football tournament which brought different services together, that drew the attention of the city council at the time:

> *we had lots of different organisations in Liverpool, so we had your abstinent organisations and you had your Salvations Armies and your hostels, which to me was just natural to do that, but when the commissioners came along to see it, they were quite blown away, because ten years ago it was very polarised, so you're either abstinent and you're on this side of the fence, or you're still using drugs and you're on this side of the fence, and there was no interaction between the two. So there was a few commissioners there from Liverpool city council who said, wow this is amazing, it really was not rocket science, it really wasn't. They seemed to think it was because they'd never seen these people mixing before. And that's how Genie was born really. They approached us then and said, look, we've seen how you've brought all these other agencies together, and how the message of recovery is being passed on to people in hostels who don't normally hear this message, and we'd like you to set something up in the centre of Liverpool, that is recovery oriented, but for people still in active addiction.*

Therefore, Genie's original aim was to provide a space for those that were on neither side of the fence, to break this polarisation between recovering and active drug users. Its 'otherness' departs from this characteristic: located in the centre of Liverpool, it constitutes a space open to those that do not feel they belong neither to strictly harm reduction nor to abstinence-based services; it is an 'other' space for those who differ from dominant classifications of active and recovering drug users. Following the event above, Genie, with the support of the city council grew fast. Initially run by volunteers, throughout the years the service managed to employ up to nine paid members of staff. The situation changed in 2016, when Liverpool city council withdrew its funding from the majority of small-scale drug and alcohol services and reallocated it to larger organisations (Clayton, Donovan and Merchant, 2016).

The specific ways in which these shifting funding practices have impacted on the caring practices provided by the services, will be addressed in the last chapter. The aim here is to draw the attention on how the historical and current relationship between the state and the provision of drug treatment, affects the daily realities of services. 18 ano, although entangled with bureaucratic and administrative apparatuses, has maintained a stable presence through its establishment as part of the national health system. Conversely, drug treatment services in the UK have historically been funded as temporary arrangements that cover certain needs for short periods of time. What this means in practice is that drug services in the UK have been dependent on the state (and subsequently the councils) for their financial survival, but never essential to it, never part of the national health system. Therefore, these small heterotopias of recovery, growing organically within cities by responding to the needs of the drug using population have always been vulnerable. They were never part of a long-term governmental funding scheme, but dependent on local councils and regularly shifting central drug treatment policies.

Along with other small-scale providers in the wider area of Merseyside, Genie lost its public funding in 2016. Inevitably, this signified changes in the daily operations of the service, including the range of the support provided to service-users, the inability of the service to keep maintaining the same number of paid members of staff, and a shift in the responsibilities of those that kept working in the service. In the account that follows, the manager of Genie narrates how the need to constantly apply for new sources of funding has affected her daily involvement with the service-users:

> *I'm a lot more desk-based than I used to be … because I used to be able to get involved a bit more on the delivery, so maybe run groups, or just being a bit more visible on the shop front if you like. And it's more back office now because there's a lot of other stuff that goes on, because we're funded by lots of different people, that means there's a lot more different reports to do and*

a lot more planning, whereas before we were just funded by more or less one person and it was just a monthly report we sent.

Genie was born out of the need to provide an alternative to the polarisation between harm reduction and recovery. While ten years ago this approach appealed to the local city council, directions coming from the central government on how drug services should be funded eventually prevailed over the needs of the drug using population. In the chapters that follow I argue that the practice of drug policy goes beyond the prioritisation of one drug treatment approach over another. However, it is important to emphasise that the shifting of the public funding from recovery-focused to harm reduction services, and the other way around, has accompanied the history of UK's drug policy. This indicates a long-term perception of people who use drugs as a homogeneous population that shares the same needs, and who can all fit under one treatment model. I will briefly address the birth of harm reduction in the UK to indicate that the involvement of the state in the way that services provide care does not only concern recovery-focused services. Whenever treatment developed in a grassroots fashion, initiated by those directly affected by drug use, the provision of public funding has been temporary and conditional, rendering treatment approaches temporal, and the services providing them vulnerable to changes and closure.

The HIV 'epidemic', and especially the threat of the virus spreading to the general population, found Thatcher's government unprepared and thus by necessity open to accept the contribution of various actors in the attempt to control the spread of the new virus. The HIV crisis provided 'a window of opportunity for different stakeholders to influence the direction of policy and practice' (Hellman, Berridge and Mold, 2016: 113). Liverpool was the first city in the UK to operate a needle exchange scheme. The programme started operating unofficially and under the government's radars in 1986, and it was not made public until 1987, when the presentation of positive outcomes was possible.

Peter McDermott (2005), part of the team that set up the first needle exchange scheme in Liverpool, argues that it was 'one handful of people' that, taking advantage of the lack of central governmental policy, created a grassroots approach of drug treatment. Unlike the voluntary organisations of the 1970s, this 'handful of people' had already secured jobs in Merseyside's health services, meaning that they were in the position to benefit from the government's inability to respond to the HIV crisis, without having to struggle for funding. In 1985 the University of Liverpool was allocated a big grant for the study of the explosion of heroin in Wirral. Around the same time, Alan Parry, an ex-heroin user from Liverpool got a job at the Mersey drug training and information centre and within 18 months in the job he got permission from his health authority manager, Howard Seymour, to set up the first needle exchange scheme. Howard Seymour was according to Russel Newcombe, who was at the time also part of the team

> *one of the suits as we call them, but underneath the suits he was fairly radical ... He basically allowed it [the needle exchange scheme] to happen, funded it, managed it, put a bit of a cloak around it to hide it, although eventually the local media were involved to get the support and to persuade the public it was a good idea*
>
> (Interview with Newcombe, November 2017)

Returning to the development of drug services as 'other' spaces, the first harm reduction initiatives of the 1980s were established as heterotopias of crisis, not only in regards to the lack of a concrete government plan, but mainly because they were practising a new way of caring for drug users. While Lifeline was originally covering nutrition and shelter needs, aspiring to become an abstinence-based TC, the first needle exchange schemes were addressing the crises of people *in* drug use, by rendering the practice of injecting safer. The success of those services cannot only be attributed to what they were providing but also to *how* they were providing it:

> *we recorded the number of needles going in and out, and it was quickly showing that nearly all of them came back and the needle exchange rate was 90 to 100%. I think partly because drug users never had people being nice to them, there was kind of a new experience for a lot of them. They'd only had criminal justice professionals and health services telling them to stop doing it or we'll put you in prison.*
>
> (Interview with Newcombe, November 2017)

This approach, driven by care and provided by people not necessarily professionally qualified, bears significant similarities to the description of Lifeline's early years. However, their histories differ in the sense that while Lifeline had to change in order to shift from a voluntary to a funded service, the first needle exchange schemes were initiated by people who were already holding positions from which they could develop those practices. Operating from that position and in combination with the 'urgency' created by the spread of HIV, allowed for the unconditional funding of the first needle exchange schemes, up until harm reduction became UK's official drug policy.

The fear for the spread of HIV to the general population, alongside the pressure coming from voluntary agencies, general practitioners and HIV activists, led to the shift of UK drug policy towards harm reduction, marked by the report of the Advisory Council on the Misuse of Drugs (ACMD), 'AIDS and Drugs Misuse' (1988). This was the first official document to acknowledge the threat of the spread of HIV as more urgent than the threat of drug use for the individual and public health. At the time, the recommendations of the report did not affect the way that harm reduction services were already operating. It just came to reaffirm, support and spread their practice. Unlike abstinence-based services, the aim of harm reduction was to approach the drug using population and attempt to reduce their risk of acquiring and spreading the HIV virus. This meant that once services could prove that they were achieving that goal they did not have to provide any other evidence to ensure the continuation of funding. Additionally, the services made sure to demonstrate how the harm reduction approach was reducing harm for the community and society and not just the drug user:

> *I think what sold it to the public wasn't just these are your sons and daughters … but also they can spread diseases to other people if they are not using these specific mechanisms.*
>
> (Interview with Newcombe, November 2017)

Retrospectively though, the AIDS and Drugs Misuse report has been regarded by some scholars as the beginning of the end of harm reduction as a grassroots movement, and the initiation of a drug policy aiming at the control and regulation of drug using bodies. Zibbel (2004) for example argues that the committee's recommendations and the new governing technologies of drug use that proceeded, do not reflect Stimson's (1983) understanding of harm reduction as a system that prioritises the drug users' rights. Conversely, it is a neoliberal approach to drug treatment that puts emphasis on individual responsibility and sidelines the responsibilities of the welfare state. This element of individual responsibility would later become the main pillar of New Labour's Third Way politics, *no rights without responsibilities* value (Giddens, 1998). At the same time, legal sanctions remained unchanged, or were increased, through what has been called 'proactive prohibition' (Measham and Moore, 2008).

Harm reduction services, the ones that had positioned the community and the drug users in the centre of attention, were eventually also affected. Although their aims were not opposed to central drug policies, they were obliged to enter the sphere of professionalisation in order to maintain their funding:

> *when the government takes over what often happens is the community gets pushed out a bit, there is a few grants thrown at the community to show that governments and local authorities have respect for them originating the policy and being involved in it but money mainly goes back to conventional drug services … just like they did with harm reduction, [it] was taken away from the community and its originators, and put in the hands of professionals some of whom, you know, are good people, others of whom really just want to do what they're told to*
>
> (Interview with Newcombe, November 2017)

The above extract echoes Yate's (1992) account on the ways the policy shift towards harm reduction affected Lifeline's mode of operation and consequently its provision of care. The concerns raised by both Newcombe and Yates go beyond their chosen treatment approaches and are more related to *how* care is provided rather than what it entails. The adoption of harm reduction by the Conservative and subsequently the New Labour party denuded it from its collective and grassroots characteristics. Instead, it was positioned in the sphere of public policy, where the focus goes beyond the minimisation of harm and focuses on the regulation of using practices and ways of being. Through the examples of Lifeline and the first harm reduction initiatives, it has been demonstrated that these policy shifts affect all services financially dependent on public and local funds. These are issues that go beyond national drug policies as well as specific treatment approaches and raise the question of how the concept and application of drug policies affects the way care is provided. Zigon (2019) describes the institutionalisation of harm reduction programs as part of the wider and international 'war on drugs' agenda:

> *In nearly every country, the drive to manage the normalized health of a working population by controlling what can and cannot be put into a body has increasingly resulted in the institutionalization of harm-reduction programs that were once organized by those people who used the drugs themselves. This has shifted what was once a political project of drug users and their allies to a state-funded therapeutic intervention run by bureaucrats, 'college-educated' managers, and public health therapists and thus largely out of the hands of drug users, who are now mostly left in the position of docile beings who must normalize or wait until they are able to do so.*
> (Zigon, 2019: 47)

For the UK the over-professionalisation[8] of services under the umbrella of specific policy instructions has rendered the work of drug-workers a bureaucratic task. Accordingly, in Greece, the bureaucratisation of the services on a higher-administrative level has left more space for drug-workers to develop therapeutic approaches but has affected their flexibility and has complicated the services' daily operation.

Genie attempted to address the polarisation between recovery and harm reduction services by creating a space for people excluded from services that apply a specific treatment approach. Although this practice drew the attention – and funding – of Liverpool city council for almost a decade, the funds were eventually redirected to larger, business-focused providers. Genie has not been the only service standing in-between harm reduction and recovery. Other empirical studies have talked about such providers as more-than-harm-reduction services (Dennis, 2019: 179), in order to address practices of care shifting from the consumption of drugs, to a concern for all the aspects of service-users' lives. I have discussed these services as heterotopias as they reflect the societies within which they emerge but are different to them. Their treatment approaches are not an application of central drug policies; they constitute other spaces for those excluded by conventional drug services. Finally, the way in which they are organised internally, the inclusions and exclusions that they create, their spatial arrangements and rules reflect Foucault's analysis of heterotopias as systems accessible to those prepared to follow certain rites and purifications. I will now expand on this last point. Having addressed the histories of 18 ano and Genie through Foucault's heterotopology, I focus on how the policymaking contexts within which they emerged have informed their current heterotopic structures.

18 ano and Genie in the Gutter: two different 'other' spaces

One of the components of the Deleuzo–Guattarian assemblage is its territoriality (Deleuze and Guattari, 2004). For the recovery assemblage this refers to the physical, but not fixed space where the recovery process takes place. Depending on the recovery programme, its services and activities, this space might take various forms (residential community, day-centre, detox centre, accommodation services, etc.), with each one of them constituting a closed, independent community with its own mode of operation. It might also be an open space, where the boundaries between the recovery assemblage and the wider community are less discerned. Such examples would be the participation of recovery programmes in community and art events. In both cases these spaces are not fixed, but always becoming through shifting affective practices. The way the territorial component of the recovery assemblage is organised also extends to the previous discussion on the recovery space as a heterotopic one. Its distance from, or proximity to other social spaces, its symbolic and physical openness, as well as the processes through which service-users are included or excluded from the recovery space, are elements that become within wider socialities and policymaking assemblages, and affect the practices of care in place.

The recovery programme of 18 ano lasts for approximately two years, and is split in three stages. The first stage has two phases: the 'consultancy station' where people can go while they are still using. The aim of that unit is to offer information about the programme, discuss the options of people considering quitting drugs and provide detoxification advice (in some cases, especially when there is a history of psychotic episodes, medication might be prescribed to deal with withdrawal symptoms). During this stage an initial assessment takes place of the social, legal and financial needs of service-users, as well as of their psychological state overall. Once a participant has managed to remain abstinent for a month, they go on to the second phase of the first stage, 'empowerment and awareness', where they start having weekly one-to-one meetings with a psychotherapist, who will remain the same throughout the duration of the programme.[9]

This first stage constitutes a heterotopia in formation. Everyone is welcome to book an appointment for an assessment, and the facilities where these appointments take place are located in the centre of Athens. As one's engagement with the heterotopia grows, the commitment towards it increases accordingly, with the main gesture, in order to gain access to the second stage of the programme, being abstinence from substances.

The second stage is called 'psychological recovery', it is inpatient and its duration is seven months. Men and women are treated separately, and one of the services is specifically designed for pregnant women and mothers with their children. During that time, service-users attend group and one-to-one psychotherapy sessions, drama therapy group and various other art groups. They are also responsible for the daily operation of the service: cooking, cleaning, financial management, etc. All these activities (communal living, personal therapy and group therapy) take place under the same roof, and during the seven months that this stage lasts service-users do not communicate with anyone outside the recovery space. This is the heterotopia par excellence: its operation as a small society reflects the 'outside', the wider context within which it emerges, while at the same time it is physically and symbolically 'elsewhere' (Foucault, 1986: 26); inaccessible to anyone who is not part of it, always belonging to those that inhabit it at the specific time, and yet temporal as the bodies that inhabit it eventually move on, and other people take their place.

Finally, the phase of social re-integration lasts for approximately one year. Group and one-to-one psychotherapy sessions continue. The participants are supported with accommodation provided by the programme, and assistance to solve any outstanding legal and health issues. It is at this stage that the heterotopia of recovery gradually returns to the wider social space from within it emerged. The services are, like in the first stage, located in the centre of the city and occasionally accessible to the service-users' families, friends and partners, when public events take place.

A concept that traverses all the stages of the programme, and the service-users become familiar with from the very beginning of their engagement with the service, is 'boundaries'. There are three main boundaries throughout all the stages of the programme: the use of substances, the use of physical and/ or verbal violence, and sexual relationships among service-users. If one or more service-users breaches them, they get automatically excluded from the heterotopia of recovery. However, this 'exclusion' does not carry the same symbolic and practical meaning in all the stages of the programme. While in the first stage, it practically means that the transition to the second stage is postponed. If a service-user though breaches one of the main boundaries while in the residential stage of the programme, they are immediately asked to leave the premises and their re-engagement with the service starts again from the first stage. Throughout the stages, this exclusion is never permanent;

nor is there a limit to the amount of times that one will be granted access to the heterotopia of recovery. However, the excluded service-user is expected to renew their commitment to the rules and boundaries of the programme through their encounters with their therapist.

Genie does not operate such a rigid system of inclusion and exclusion. Conversely, it focuses on *managing* boundaries *within* the heterotopic space. This differentiation between the services is associated with the specific territorialities of the two assemblages, as well as with the policymaking, political and social contexts within which they were established. Genie is a drug and alcohol recovery-focused daily service. The service-users are not expected to maintain abstinence but to present in a state that they are able to participate in group discussions and to show a certain level of commitment towards recovery – this mainly means that they are expected to manage and/or gradually reduce their drug and alcohol intake. These organisational and structural differences to 18 ano are also the ones that define the ways in which the heterotopic space is produced. While in the case of 18 ano, one of the main pillars that leads to the inclusion or exclusion of service-users from the recovery space is abstinence, the fact that Genie is open to people that are using, renders the gestures that ensure access to the heterotopia of recovery fluid and negotiable. Unlike the boundaries of 18 ano that extend beyond the recovery space – as maintaining abstinence does not only refer to the time service-users spend in the premises of recovery – the rules of Genie are solely focused on the time the service-user spends *inside* the recovery space, and do not extend beyond it.

From differences to connections

The histories of 18 ano and Genie have been addressed in relation to their formation as heterotopias within specific policymaking contexts. Going beyond specific treatment approaches, the aim has been to historicise treatment practices by accounting for their emergence as 'other spaces'. 18 ano was produced as a heterotopia of crisis, 'other' to the psychiatric and bureaucratic system of thought on which it remains dependent but also in conflict with. Genie was born within a tradition of flowing, transitory, precarious and temporal (Foucault, 1986: 28) services, constantly balancing between their grassroots origin and shifting policy demands. Through Foucault's heterotopology, I have addressed the contingent historical identity that constitutes each recovery assemblage an individual entity (DeLanda, 2016). In the chapters that follow, I stay with the Deleuzo–Guattarian assemblage to address the becomings of the service-users with and without drugs, as well as the becoming affective encounters increasing a body's capacity to act. This analysis moves beyond the historical structural differences of the collaborating services, and focuses on the connections made possible between the two assemblages, and beyond them.

Notes

1 United Nations Office on Drugs and Crime (2020) www.unodc.org/unodc/en/treaties/

2 Chiara Strutti was part of a six member-team of Franco Rotelli, that were at the time visiting the psychiatric hospitals of Greece to make suggestions for the de-institutionalisation of the 'institutions of violence' (Matsa, in the preface of 'Leros to La Borde', 2015: 11).

3 £2,50.

4 For more information on this issue see KETHEA (2019) www.kethea.gr/en/nea/vote-for-the-autonomy-kethea-therapeutic-communities/

5 HMSO (1926). Report of the Departmental Committee on Morphine and Heroin Addiction. Ministry of Health.

6 HMSO (1965). Drug Addiction: The Second Report of the Interdepartmental Committee. Ministry of Health.

7 The information on Genie's history comes from my interview with Carolyn Edwards.

8 It can also be argued that the same policies have led to the de-professionalisation of services, through the mobilisation of 'recovery champions', who are volunteers leading recovery groups with no pay and little recognition or support (Measham, Moore and Welch, 2013).

9 www.18ano.gr/

Chapter 5

Becoming a drug user – becoming a service-user

I felt like it all fell into place, everything changed from that day onwards[1]

The 'drug assemblage' has been empirically and analytically deployed to explore the human and non-human encounters that bring the drug event into being (Bøhling, 2015; Dennis, 2016; Dilkes-Frayne, 2014; Dilkes-Frayne and Duff, 2017). The primary aim of these studies has been to challenge moralising and normalising frames of thought that produce substance users as flawed and disempowered subjectivities. Mobilising the 'drug assemblage' has opened up a path for innovative approaches to harm reduction, where the question of pleasure is not sidelined, but positioned in the focus of attention (Bøhling, 2017; Dennis, 2019).

In line with the theoretical framework of this body of work, my initial question has been what happens when we shift our empirical gaze from the narratives and lived experiences of active drug users to those engaging with recovery; to those that at some point identified their use as problematic, and made the decision to either abstain or change their ways of using. How is pleasure, desire and its memory renegotiated and how can these narratives inform policymaking beyond harm reduction? This shifting empirical gaze has given birth to this book's commitment to bring the drug assemblage within the recovery assemblage; to follow the becomings of subjects from substance users to service-users and to unravel how the flows of care that take place in the recovery assemblage render this transition possible.

I do so by following the narratives of people in recovery on their first experiences of drug use, the time that drug use was part of their daily lives, and their engagement with services, occasionally interrupted by relapses or other events. Unlike studies primarily concerned with the minimisation of harm, I am not looking how the drug event can be 'done better' (Dennis, 2019). I am not looking for the 'good' and 'bad' encounters that take place *within the drug assemblage*, but how these experiences are reflected upon *within the recovery assemblage*, as well as how existing recovery practices respond

DOI: 10.4324/9781003165613-6

to drug using experiences. This way of thinking empirically with people in recovery becomes possible through McLeod's (2017) empirical research on wellbeing. McLeod's *wellbeing machine* is not only constituted of positive and hopeful experiences. Becoming-well is not a linear story where the wellness gradually and steadily prevails over the illness, but a complicated one where wellbeing becomes possible through illbeing; where de-stratification, the inability to pull a self together and the associated affective states of despair and immobilisation (2017: 125) are essential and inextricable parts of the wellbeing assemblage. Following McLeod, I take participants' encounters with drugs and the interruptions of their recovery process seriously. I am interested in the recovery encounters that these experiences render possible; the practices of care that resist policymaking discourses that frame as 'failures' any diversions from a linear route. Conversely, I approach these destratifications as components of the becoming-well process. This frame of thought is in alliance with Murphy's call for the unsettlement of care (2015), a better politics of care that does not conflate it with sympathy, attachment and positive feelings as political goods, but a troubling care that works against hegemonic structures (Murphy, 2015: 719). In what follows it is demonstrated how the complexity and non-linearity of wellbeing (McLeod, 2017) is addressed through the becoming of an affectively charged protocol of recovery (Murphy, 2015). This protocol opposes hegemonic structures by resisting the production of 'recovered', fixed and stable subjectivities and enables instead subjectivities to unfold in all their complexity. These entanglements are produced and held together by the service-users' *desire of becoming-other*, the desire to connect, the desire to live otherwise. The power of the recovery assemblage lies in its potentiality to enable the re-emergence of the repressed desire, to work towards its expansion (Colebrook, 2001: 91), to support the enhancement of life.

Becoming a drug user

Rather than a policy approach or a treatment model, the recovery assemblage is explored as the caring response to those whose substance intake has shifted from a line of flight to a line of death (Deleuze and Guattari, 2004: 314). It does not come into being in a void, but in relation and in response to the using experiences of those that inhabit it. I start from the participants' first experiences of substance use; from their attempt to make sense of these past experiences, as recovering subjects in the present. In these accounts the relationship between the recovering subject and the substance is complicated and under negotiation. The narratives of people in recovery come into being at a time when they feel that the destratifications associated with substance use override the potentiality of deterritorialisations, leading to the production of reflexive and emotionally informed stories. Self-reflection in that sense is an intrinsic component of the voluntary engagement with the recovery process, a process that involves a telling, a re-storying of one's life. The narratives that follow emerge from the encounter between the questions asked and the service-users as they were *becoming with the recovery assemblage.*

Accounts of people in recovery occasionally reflect the binary and moralising discourses within which they are historically becoming. Within this framework drug use is by default associated with a chaotic lifestyle and sobriety with wellbeing –

> *I've got a good routine now as well, so I go – I wake up early, get ready to come here [Genie], I'm out all day, and then I go to sleep early, whereas when I was on drugs, my sleeping pattern was very chaotic, yeah, I'll be awake for days, I'll be sleeping for days, it was bad, but it's good now.*

However, the recovery assemblage, a safe space where reflection, negotiation and doubt are enhanced, also opens up a potentiality for the narration of stories where the memory of pleasure remains strong and present:

> *Oh it's very powerful! It's very strong, very strong, you know, all your face goes all tingly you know and your fingers go all swollen and tingly and your feet and everything you know, and then you think you go [breathes out] and then you're surrounded by pillows or something, you know, you're surrounded by clouds or something like that, and a soft, soft existence, it's very strange. So anyway, the next day I went out and bought a syringe! And everything! So I thought, ooh I'm going to try some more of this. So then I started injecting … And after that it never stopped until about let's see, it's 2018, I think I took it till about 2015, no, say 2012.*

Even in cases when abstinence has either not been achieved or not been set as a target, pleasure is occasionally acknowledged without shame or guilt:

> *I mean there are things I can do you know to avoid that, but I choose not to, I choose to have a drink. And to be perfectly honest with you, I do it because I enjoy it as well, but I know now as well if it's going too far, if it's getting out of hand, that's when I'll know.*

Such accounts only reflect a specific understanding of pleasure, a single aspect of a complicated term that 'is notoriously difficult to define and there is little consensus about what it is or how it works' (Race, 2017: 145). Empirical drug and alcohol scholars have researched pleasure, thought about it and most recently thought *with* pleasure (Race, 2017: 145). Through a close examination of the narrations of first experiences of drug use, the difficulty to grasp pleasure, its meaning and experience has become apparent, as it is not always constructed in contradiction with, but occasionally goes hand in hand with suffering.

> *with the smack I threw up but I liked so much the way I was feeling ... It was like I was seeing myself up in the sky and I'm like, such peacefulness, such warmth, where am I gonna find that again. And although I suffered then, I was vomiting for a week, what I was feeling in that moment, I wouldn't have changed it for the world back then.*

Accounts where suffering and pleasure do not just coexist but co-constitute the using experience overall, resonate with findings of empirical studies where uncomfortable feelings are identified as indicators that the drug injection has been 'successful' (Dennis, 2019: 84). They also empirically demonstrate that drugs enable differentiations and transformations of the body that are not necessarily or directly pleasurable (Malins, 2017: 129). Therefore, I have chosen to address the ambivalence associated with first experiences of drug use by thinking with desire, rather than with pleasure. Following Deleuze and Guattari (2004), I argue that the motivation for 'risk-taking' activities cannot be captured when thought of as an attempt to achieve pleasure and pain (Malins, 2017: 130). Conversely, these feelings are components of assemblages that bodies mobilise in their attempts to enable desire to flow (ibid.). Thinking first experiences of drug use with desire paves the way for the comprehension of the relationship between a subject and a substance as a complex situational interaction (Oksanen, 2013: 61) driven by the need to enable the flow of desire.

In 'Desire and Pleasure' (Deleuze, 2007), originally a letter addressed to Michel Foucault in 1977 after the publication of the first volume of *History of Sexuality* (1990), Deleuze attempts to make a distinction between the two terms:

> *The last time we saw each other, Michel [Foucault] kindly and affection-ately told me something like the following: 'I can't stand the word desire; even if you use it differently, I can't stop myself from thinking or experien-cing the fact that desire = lack, or that desire is repressed' ... For one thing, I can barely stand the word pleasure ... For me, desire includes no lack; it is also not a natural given. Desire is wholly a part of functioning heteroge-neous assemblage. It is a process, as opposed to a structure or a genesis. It is an affect, as opposed to a feeling ... Pleasure seems to me to be on the side of strata and organization ... Pleasure seems to me to be the only means for persons or subjects to orient themselves in a process that exceeds them. It is a re-territorialization.*
>
> (2007: 130–131)

Deleuze's understanding of desire as a process rather than a structure, as an affect rather than a feeling, is useful for our understanding of the narratives of first experiences of drug use. Although pleasure has been accounted for as affect (Bøhling, 2017) producing 'new subjectivities and becomings rather than being an end point, a closing down of affect' (Dennis, 2019: 19), it still refers to the specific affective relations produced between the encounter of a subject with a substance. Mobilising desire, my attempt is to account for *the becomings* desired *through* the substance, rather than the desire *for* the substance.

The Deleuzian becoming does not have 'an origin or being that then becomes or goes through a process of simulation ... there "is" nothing other than the flow of becoming' (Colebrook, 2001: 125). There is no distinction of past and future either; becoming moves and pulls in both directions at once, fragmenting the subject following this double direction (Deleuze, 1990: 1–3). Like desire, becoming is a process and there is no origin or interpretation of a body's desired becomings; it is simply 'a desire to expand or become other through what is more than oneself' (Colebrook, 2001: 134–135). Material bodies are thus defined in part by reference to the ways in which they can become-other. This modification becomes possible when they act upon other bodies or when they are acted upon by other bodies (Patton, 2000: 78). Desire is the machine that drives these modifications, 'the affects and intensities that correspond to a body's relations with other bodies' (ibid.: 78–79), enhancing or blocking its capacity to act.

Following the narratives of first experiences of drug use, I look at the service-users' desire of becoming-other; the desire to experiment with what the body can do, or to make the body function better or differently (Malins, 2017: 130). I then move on to explore how the recovery assemblage responds to the desire of becoming-other by replacing the affects produced by drugs with affective relations produced through practices of care.

Becoming Loved
First time I used it was hash. With a guy I was supposed to be in love. Also [he was] my first sexual relationship. In a house where there was a couple, also supposed to be in love and it instantly crossed my mind that that's how love is, something that I didn't have in my life ... That's love and that's how I can experience it. A big gap that I had would be filled. And a great need. And that's how it went with me and drugs. That's what I thought.

Becoming part of
It [drug use] made me feel like I belong. Nothing more. Lots of times I didn't like what I was doing but the fact that I belonged to a group that did something, for me was very important. And made me feel special and stronger ...

I grew up without my father ... my mother didn't have much time cause she was working so in a way I was dissatisfied at home. You can't understand [at that age] how dissatisfied you are but you know inside you that it's not easy for you to become part of a group cause you've been lonely growing up. In school you're expected to become part of a group and you don't even know how to become accepted. That [using drugs] was a way for me to become accepted.

Becoming care-free
It was the absolute relief from anxieties, from anything that bothered me that time, heartbreaks, my studies that I didn't like at all, my relationship with my family. I mean I was taking the pills and I was going out there and my relationship with the world was completely transformed ... I felt like a feather, so light physically and emotionally.

The accounts above complicate the question of desire. The Deleuzian desire 'does not begin from lack – desiring what we do not have. Desire begins from connection; life strives to preserve and enhance itself and does so by connecting with other desires' (Colebrook, 2001: 91). These service-users' first experiences of drug use express both a lack of and a desire for physical and emotional connections with another body, with a group, with the world. Mediated by a substance, they talk about their desires and first encounters with drugs as the beginnings of destratifications.

Whether this is a destratified desire or not, it is not against life; it is a desire for the expansion of life through creation and transformation (Colebrook, 2001: 135). Katerina Matsa, psychiatrist, director of 18 ano for many years and one of the people that established the programme's therapeutic practice, famously used to say (as discussed in the interviews with recovery workers from 18 ano) that 'people do not take drugs because they want to die; they take them because they want to live'. They are not looking for pleasure, but for becomings that will expand the possibilities of life. The above accounts show just that; a desire to find a way to live, to become loved, part-of and care-free. They are not imaginary aspirations of 'another' life, but rather productions of realities enabled by the active force of desire (Oksanen, 2013: 60). And yet, according to Katerina Matsa, to the service workers I interviewed in Athens and Liverpool, to the service-users engaging with recovery, and also according to Deleuze and Guattari, when the desire of becoming-other is mediated by substances, it eventually gets destratified and blocked. Deleuze and Guattari's writings on drugs are not extensive, and in many cases controversial (Malins, 2004). Their intervention though is useful and contributes to our current discussion on the desire of becoming-other through drugs.

Two questions on drugs: causality and the turning point

Deleuze identifies two questions that require contemplation in our thinking with drugs. 'The first question would be: Do drugs have a *specific causality* and can we explore this direction?' (2007: 151, emphasis in original). The same question is addressed in *A Thousand Plateaus* (2004). In both these texts the causality of drugs entails a desire for deterritorialisation, the perception of the imperceptible (Deleuze and Guattari, 2004: 311). Deleuze and Guattari write about drugs having in mind the drug experiences of the beat generation, the experimentations of Antonin Artaud with peyote and Henri Michaux with mescaline. They are interested in exploring where and how the plane of drugs collapses:

> *The causal line, or the line of flight, of drugs is constantly being segmentarized … The deterritorializations remain relative, compensated for by the most abject reterritorializations, so that the imperceptible and perception continually pursue or run after each other without ever truly coupling. Instead of holes in the world allowing the world lines themselves to run off, the lines of flight coil and start to swirl in black holes; to each addict a hole, group or individual, like a snail. Down, instead of high.*
>
> (Deleuze and Guattari, 2004: 314)

The question of causality is addressed here in relation to a different source of data. The writings of Michaux, Artaud, the beatniks and others are testimonies of their desire to become bodies without organs; an exploration of a body's capacity to act beyond social norms and connections. And although the failures of their bodies through these attempts can be read in parallel with the physical and emotional sufferings of people that identify as addicts, the accounts shared above of first experiences of drug use reveal another causality and a different desire; the desire of becoming-other *within* a given social environment. These accounts of desires of becoming loved, becoming part of and becoming care-free are not desires for transcendental but for mundane, daily experiences. Deleuze and Guattari are interested in drugs as modifications of speed (2004). The positive experience of drugs is associated with an acceleration that makes 'holes in the world allowing the world lines themselves to run off' (Deleuze and Guattari, 2004: 314). Eventually this line of flight becomes a line of death when the speed fades out and the body of the user slows down, starting to swirl in black holes, like a snail (ibid.). Conversely, some of the service-users' first experiences of drug use were *about* slowing down, reducing speed and becoming light: '*I felt like a feather, so light physically and emotionally*'. The complexity of the production of time with drugs, as well as the relationship between drugs, movement and immobility have been part of Olievenstein's analysis of the understanding of the drug using subjectivity:

> *A boy or a girl consuming drugs, accesses indeed an erupted time, where they experience truly unbelievable accelerating and decelerating phenomena. One minute might feel like a fracture of a second or, the other way around, a whole year. The drug user, in one moment, can get an enlightening*

perspective of their whole life, and of the phantasies that govern it; they will discover, in some kind of explosion, everything that various years of psychoanalysis would have laboriously tried to unveil. But on the other hand, they will sometimes hear the tic-tac of a clock taking them to infinity ... The space of the drug users is not less twisted and distorted. They sometimes have the feeling that they are elsewhere, that they traverse various worlds, that they 'fly', that they 'live in another planet', according to their own terminology. Other times though, they are seized by a true vertigo of immobility and they stay for whole hours nailed in bed. Finally, sometimes, a drunkenness of speed takes them away, they are always in the process of moving, running, obsessed by the need for a change of place.

(Olievenstein, 1977: 190)

In this quote acceleration and deceleration alternate, making new connections possible and then blocking them again. Space is also expanded and diminished, leading to a state of immobility or endless mobility. Issues of temporality and specifically the desire of becoming-slow will be addressed later (*Beyond the recovery assemblage: deterritorialisation and reterritorialisation*). My aim here in response to Deleuze's call for an exploration of the drugs' causality is to emphasise that causality should be addressed *through and with the empirical*. Following the lived experiences of people in recovery challenges attempts for the provision of generalised interpretations and assumptions about the desires that drive drug use, and emphasises the complexity of the drug event.

Exploring a specific causality is not a process of trying to form a linear connection between the use of a substance and a cause, but to map the territory or contours of a drug set (Deleuze, 2007: 151). The experiences shared do just that. The focus of those narratives is not on characters or objects, but on environments and desires. It is not the substance that matters, but the becomings that become possible through it – becoming loved, becoming part of, becoming care-free. Pleasure is either not present or not accounted for. In the becoming-loved narrative the service-user later on described the experience as a 'very ugly' one:

And after I smoked [the hash] I was a mess. I had sat on a chair. I couldn't move. I'll never forget that moment. I was all numb and heavy. That's what I remember from the first time [I used drugs]. Very ugly experience.

The substance in this account is not used for pleasure but as a means to fulfil the desire of becoming-loved ('*that's how love is*'). Accordingly, in the first 'becoming part of' narrative, the service-user '*lots of times didn't like what [she] was doing*'. While the corporeal modifications associated with the use of substances are both positive and negative, the emphasis in these narratives is on the relations and connections becoming through the substance; the assemblages produced allowing for the desire to flow. '*The fact that I belonged to a group that did something, for me was very important'*, the participant says, shifting the attention from the drug, to the socialities produced around it. Finally, in the second 'becoming part of' and the 'becoming care-free' account, the drug is again talked about as the key for the flow of desires – becoming acceptable, becoming light, becoming social – rather than as a pleasurable device in itself.

Thinking first experiences of drug use with desire goes beyond the desire *for* drugs and brings into the picture the desire *of becoming-other*. While for some service-users, first experiences of drug use were associated with pleasure – or the negotiation between suffering and pleasure, in the accounts shared above it is the territory of the drug set that is positioned in the focus of attention. Following these accounts, looking for the causality of drug use is not about looking for 'a cause and effect' structure; it is a process that carefully follows the desired becomings that drug use enables. Deleuze and Guattari hoped that following causality could potentially lead to the golden ratio of drug use:

> *To succeed in getting drunk, but on pure water (Henri Miller). To succeed in getting high, but by abstention … To reach the point where 'to get high or not to get high' is no longer the question, but rather whether drugs have sufficiently changed the general conditions of space and time perception so that nonusers can succeed in passing through the holes in the world and following the lines of flight at the very place where means other than drugs become necessary.*
>
> (Deleuze and Guattari, 2004: 315)

Following the causality of becoming-other though leads to another direction, the beginning of the identification of the blocked desires that eventually rendered drug use essential. Following this line of thought, the substance is not perceived as an object of desire but as an agent of becoming (Deleuze and Guattari, 2004: 313). 'Addiction' according to the two philosophers happens when the desire for drugs fundamentally alters the desiring production and prevails over all other assemblages, narrowing down the possibilities in life (Oksanen, 2013: 61). Deleuze's second question on drugs addresses the specific causality of this transition: the causality of what he calls the 'turning point'; the moment when active lines of flight roll up and turn into black holes; dug in instead of spaced out (Deleuze, 2007: 153). Deleuze's turning point is when vital experimentation turns into deadly experimentation, when 'all control is lost and the system of abject dependence begins' (ibid.). Claude Olievenstein's (1977) definition of addiction, together with the narrations of people in recovery will help us account for this 'turning point'.

Olievenstein defines addiction as the encounter between a certain substance and an individual, at a very specific moment in that person's life. In other words, it is the encounter between an object and a subject in a time and a place that can change everything and make it all *'fall into place'*, as said by one of the participants, quoted at the very beginning of this chapter. This affective encounter escapes any attempts for generalisations, as its uniqueness renders it unpredictable. The uniqueness of this encounter lays in the fact that it does not refer to *any* individual, *any* substance and *any given time*, but has very *specific* material and immaterial components that need to come together for Deleuze's turning point to happen:

> *I'd been hospitalised due to a mental breakdown ... Coming out from there, there was this guy I knew, he'd brought me a joint. I didn't like it, I had tried weed and cocaine a few times before, nothing crazy, and anyway I didn't smoke the joint. After some time he brought me cocaine, and although I had used [cocaine] before, that time was different, that night was different. I mean, the moment I used I'm like 'here we are', at least for a while until I get better cause I had depression, I was in a bad state and I said [I'll use] for a bit until I'm better, I mean, how joyful and light I felt. And all the anxieties were gone.*

The accounts of first experiences of drug use discussed earlier were narratives of processes, of the use of drugs as an agent of becoming-other. The narrative above is also an account of a first experience of drug use, talked about as *a rupture in time*; not the first time that drugs were being used, but the first time that drug use *made sense* in a specific way. The link between these two types of narratives of experiences of drug use is their investment with the desire of becoming-other, and specifically the desire of becoming-light, a desire that flows when a person (the narrator with all the memories she carries) meets a substance (cocaine) at a specific moment in time (right after having been hospitalised for a mental health issue). This is an application of Claude Olievenstein's definition of addiction and a response that complicates Deleuze's second question on drugs, how do we account for the turning point.

As described by Deleuze, the turning point happens when drug use shifts from a vital connection to a line of death. However, the service-users' narratives account for more complex turning points; experiences where drug use renders the desired becoming-other possible, moments in time when a becoming destratification takes the shape and form of deterritorialisation. Dennis (2019) argues that the 'turning point', as deployed by Deleuze, cannot account for the shift from becoming-other to becoming-blocked. Following Malins (2004), she claims that these narratives are better conceived of as stratifications, rather than destratifications or disconnections (Dennis, 2019: 115). My aim is to demonstrate that the 'turning point' should not be dismissed, but re-worked in a Deleuzian and Guattarian way. There is an ambivalence inherent in all of the two philosophers' concepts; nothing is unambiguously good or bad (Patton, 2000: 66). Accordingly, based on service-users' accounts, the 'turning point' is much more than a shift of a line of flight to a line of death. When asking for reflections on first encounters with substances, the narrations were not primarily concerned with whether the story told was actually about the first time that one used drugs. The first time was rather understood as *this* time; the time that drugs made sense in a *different* way and '*it all fell into place*'. This is what I refer to as the 'turning point', an ambivalent – in the Deleuzo–Guattarian sense – figure, neither good nor bad, but powerful enough to account for the shifts in a person's becoming with a drug.

Going back to Dennis's (2019) argument for stratifications instead of destratifications when accounting for the shift from becoming-other to becoming-blocked, I have chosen to follow McLeod (2017) (theoretically) and my participants' accounts (empirically) and to take destratifications seriously. Taking into consideration the fact that the narratives shared here come from people in recovery, the time when '*it all fell into place*' is more often than not followed by the time when it all went wrong. In that sense, turning points are accounted for as destratifications in the shape and form of deterriotrialisations. The main prerogative here is to explore how these narratives come to shape the recovering practices of care, rather than to account for underexplored connections and stratifications within the drug encounter. McLeod's work shows 'how suffering, illbeing and sad passions are essential elements in the dynamic experience of health' (McLeod, 2017: 154). Instead of looking for the connections or stratifications within the drug assemblage, I focus on the 'cracks' (Deleuze, 1990) and destratifications and how these are addressed and incorporated in the recovery assemblage.

Turning points are empirical ways to understand the becomings that traverse drug use and recovery. They are talked about as ruptures with time, moments when drugs made sense. This time and space specific turning point, does not happen in isolation and in a random fashion. As described by Olievenstein (1977) it is the outcome of a very specific encounter at a given time between a subject and a substance, and it carries a causality that can be accounted for through the becomings desired by the service-users, even before their encounter with the substance. Accounted for in all their complexity, turning points guide our unfolding of the process of becoming a drug user, leading to another set of turning points, the decision to interrupt or change the relationship with a substance, the desire of becoming a service-user. This is a path carrying its own disruptions and ruptures, but before moving on, I want to return to the complexity of the turning point, sharing a narrative where the substance is not even present.

I mean I used to drink socially, you know which was like pretty normal for like a lad of my age, you know with your mates, weekends and what have you, and you just go out, but it was never a problem. But my problems really began when my mother died, she died on my twenty sixth birthday and I was really close to my mum, and it hit me really hard that, and I just couldn't seem to deal with it, I could not, I just wanted to try and escape from it all and my way of going about escaping and blocking it or avoiding whatever was going on was just, I turned to alcohol, and that just progressed ... I suppose that really kicked in before my mum died, it could have been because of the circumstances when my dad died, as I mentioned to you he was a chronic alcoholic and he killed himself when I was fifteen, and this was during the summer holidays, leading into my last year in school, you know, exams and everything, so there was a lot going on, and that really affected me so much, but I didn't really deal with it or talk about it to any-body, I just kept that with me. But I know it changed me, I could feel the change within myself, you know, my confidence was shattered really, it was like I was trying to be what I used to be but it wasn't working because I was putting the effort in, it just wasn't like a natural thing the way it used to be for me. So yeah, I think that's when it all started, you know, the thoughts and everything.

The account above begins with the narration of the shift from drinking socially to drinking problematically, the turning point that takes place when the narrator consumes alcohol after the death of his mother, driven by the desire to become emotionally blocked. As the narration continues, a second turning point comes into being. The event here is the death of the father at a time that '*there was a lot going on*'. Unlike the previous accounts, the sub-stance here is only indirectly present: '*as I mentioned to you he [the dad] was a chronic alcoholic*', but the affect of the event is strongly acknowledged: '*I know it changed me, I could feel the change within myself, you know*'. This takes us back to the previous discussion on the exploration of causality as a mapping of the territory of the drug set, the context within a desire emerges; not the desire for the drug itself but the desire of becoming-other. Becoming loved, becoming care-free, becoming light, becoming part of and, as discussed in the account above, becoming-blocked are desires emerging in assemblages where the substance is not necessarily the protagonist. Its presence however does render the desired becomings possible, before these get blocked, as the sub-stance gradually occupies more and more space and time, diminishing rather than enhancing the possibilities of life.

All these narratives are answers to the question 'Could you talk to me about the first time you used?' accompanied by questions on the feelings associated with that experience and the environments where it took place. The stories told are not suitable for the production of generalisations on first experiences of drug use. They are not even strictly first experiences of drug use, but accounts of the first time that drugs made sense in a specific way. They are testimonies of the uniqueness and complexity that accompany the initial encounter of a subject with a substance. For some of the service-users the driving force of their narratives has been pleasure: nostalgia of the feeling of the first hit, mixed with descriptions of the first corporeal suffering associated with drug use. The second set of accounts addressed causality and the desire of becoming-other, and the third accounted for the turning point and the desire of becomimg-light and emotionally blocked. For the two latter sets of narratives it is not the substance itself that is positioned in the focus of attention, but the desires invested in the drug use experience.

The aim of the exploration of first experiences of drug use has not been to look for similarities, but for the uniqueness of each and every one of these experiences. The majority of the current policy documents call for individualised care packages and tailor-made recovery approaches that would respond to the needs of each individual. However, there is a lack of further explanations on what this individualised treatment entails. My attempt has been to demonstrate that any form of care that rejects generalisations should have as a starting point the narratives of the person that at a given time in their life asks for help. This way of thinking about policy reflects Mol's (2008) call for a shift from a logic of choice to a logic of care. Thinking with care requires time, attention and a renegotiation of terms and their meanings. Tracing the desires associated with drug use, as the service-users narrate them, is a way to take their lived experiences and needs seriously. The acknowledgment of 'turning points' in the relationship of a subject with the substance is also moving towards the same direction.

By focusing on how the service-users talk about the transitions and the becomings that are enabled or blocked from the first encounter with the substance, to drug use as a daily practice, and to the first encounter with recovery services, my aim is twofold: (a) to account for the uniqueness of each using experience and therefore challenge homogenising approaches about the causality of drug use, which do not take into consideration the specific desires that drug use addresses, and (b) to argue that the desire that brings all these experiences together is a desire for connection, a desire for care unpacked in the chapters that follow. Rather than perceiving drugs as inherently bad through a pharmacological and medicalised gaze, thinking with desire goes beyond the corporeal impacts of substances, and traces the desired life possibilities that first experiences of use were able to enhance. Accounting for turning points explores the specific connections desired, the connections that as we will see later on, the recovery assemblage is called to enhance and establish, by replacing the use of substances with the provision of care.

Finally, this is also an attempt to respond to the debate on the distinction between dependent and recreational use, the transition from one form of use to another (Askew, 2016; Decorte, 2001; Rhodes et al., 2011), as well as to challenge the view that researchers and policymakers have to 'choose' between harm reduction and recovery approaches. By focusing on lived experiences of drug use and recovery, we can shift the focus of attention from medicalised approaches of drug use, primarily concerned with the classification of substances and the regulation of drug use, to the connections that the encounter between a subjectivity and a substance render possible. The last two narratives show that a distinction between addictive and non-addictive substances, and quests for the ideal frequency and amount of use, fail to appreciate the complexity of the drug encounter. In both these cases service-users had been 'recreational' users before identifying their use as problematic, a shift that occurred not because of a change from a 'soft' to a 'hard' drug, but through complex life experiences, thoughts, practices and desires that rendered the 'turning point' possible. This resonates with Dennis's empirical findings which demonstrate that pleasure is not enough for the distinction between 'recreational' and 'addictive' use, on the contrary it blocks the service-users' attempts to make sense of their practices (2019: 59). It also reflects Malins's argument that the binary distinction between pleasurable and painful experiences cannot fully account for the things that unsettle us, provoke or transform us (2017: 130). Being attentive to drug users' accounts while thinking with the desire of becoming-other opens up another way of talking about recreational and problematic use, beyond moralising discourses, mainly concerned with the regulation of pleasure. '... for Deleuze and Guattari the possibility of becoming-other is indeed present at every moment. It is realised in those moments when a qualitatively different kind of transition is involved' (Patton, 2000: 85). Following Deleuze and Guattari, I argue that drug use becomes 'dependent' or 'problematic' when the substances, instead of augmenting a body's capacity to act, block its desire of becoming-other, an experience that can only be accounted for as destratified by the users themselves.

In what follows I go back to narratives of drug use, focusing now on the time that drug use had become an essential part of the service-users' daily lives. These accounts will be closely explored through the question of desire, freedom and time.

Drug use as everyday practice

Following the service-users' first experiences of drug use it has been argued that thinking solely with pleasure cannot fully account for the complexity of these experiences and their entanglement with suffering and hope for the enhancement of the possibilities of life. Desire, conversely, allows us to explore the connections enabled through the substance and the anticipated becomings the subject attempts to achieve. Staying with desire and the ambivalence of the drug use event, I now focus on the time that drug use was established as an everyday practice in the service-users' lives, introducing into this daily encounter between the subject and the substance the question of freedom. Through empirical accounts I argue for a needed disassociation between the 'freedom to make healthy choices' and the 'freedom to become other', before moving on to suggest that, in relation to drug use, freedom (and the lack of it) is better understood as a question of time, rather than morality. Drawing on the writings of Fitzgerald (1945) and Lowry (1965) with alcohol, Deleuze says that *alcoholism does not seem to be a search for pleasure, but a search for an effect which consists mainly in an extraordinary hardening of the present … alcohol is at once love and the loss of love, money and the loss of money, the native land and its loss. It is at once object, loss of object, and the law governing this loss within an orchestrated process of demolition.*

(Deleuze, 1990: 158–160, emphasis in original)

Deleuze's understanding of alcoholism reflects the complexity of the empirical accounts of the initial and habitual encounters between the subjects and the substances. This encounter is not talked about as 'good' or 'bad'; it is both, simultaneously enabling and blocking desires, at *once love and the loss of love, an object and the loss of it.* Taking the ambivalence that accompanies drug use seriously and thinking with desire, opens the way for the understanding of freedom not as a stable and fixed end-point that is either achieved or lost, but as a process, a desire looking for ways to flow, *the desire of becoming-free.* This understanding of freedom clashes with its neoliberal definition as the ability and moral responsibility to make 'healthy and responsible choices', a thought process that constitutes daily drug use as the opposite to freedom. Conversely, it resonates with an understanding of freedom 'as an openness to possibilities by which one lets worlds and their inhabitants become what they may, free of the imposition and control of categories and normalization' (Zigon, 2019: 105).

Helen Keane (2002) has critically followed the historical and cultural construction of addiction as the antithesis of freedom and how this contributes to the neoliberal production of human beings as autonomous individuals, governed and defined through a certain notion of freedom. Within this context addiction is framed as a pathological inability to exercise self-control and ambivalence is regarded as proof of an individual's weakness to make the 'right' choice. O'Malley and Valverde's (2004) analysis follows the shifts in the relationship between pleasure and freedom from liberal to neoliberal times. By the end of the 19th century, drug users' freedom was rendered problematic and their pleasure pathological, reflecting the emergence of the 'free' subject under liberal governance (O'Malley and Valverde, 2004: 27). Under neoliberalism, lifestyle and choice become the new ways of exercising freedom in the world of the 'sovereign consumer', and the compulsion of addiction transforms accordingly into a freedom of choice, rendering individuals personally responsible for the governance of harm (ibid.: 36–39). Studies that pathologise drug use have, wittingly or unwittingly, contributed to the construction of drug use as antithetical to freedom. Accordingly, damage-centred research, solely documenting pain and loss and thinking of drug users as broken (Tuck, 2009) does little to account for the complexity of drug use and the desires of becoming associated with it.

The empirical account that follows demonstrates this complexity and challenges the neoliberal construction of freedom as the ability to make 'healthy' choices. Alternatively, it positions in the focus of attention the ambivalence and the desire of becoming-free, a desire that in this case clashes with dominant perceptions of health:

> *I started asking the girls [sex workers] at Vathis square how they felt working with the clients, [I told them that] I can't be home anymore, I can't stand this pressure, I want my mother to know what's going on and [I want to] feel more free … The past few years I was staying on the street and at Pedio to Areos, I stayed at Menidi*[2] *too, in abandoned buildings, in clients' houses, on benches, and yet* I liked that too back then.

> (my emphasis)

Freedom in this account is discussed in relation to the desire to get disassociated from one assemblage – the maternal home – and produce another – the drug assemblage. While from a neoliberal perspective home-lessness and the engagement with 'risky activities' like sex work are anti-thetical to freedom, in the account above they constitute the means through which freedom becomes possible. Retrospectively, the service-user herself is surprised by her past practices, not because of their identification as risky but because at the time they were identified as pleasurable ('*and yet I liked that too back then*'). And yet there is no indication that the choices made back then were wrong. Returning to Deleuze, the question that arises is not whether there is enough knowledge available about what a 'healthy' choice is, but whether sometimes the health given is not what one desires:

> *If one asks why health does not suffice, why the crack is desirable, it is per-haps because only by means of the crack and at its edges thought occurs, that anything that is good and great in humanity enters and exits through it, in people ready to destroy themselves – better death than the health which we are given.*

> (Deleuze, 1990: 160)

What the service-user rejects is not health overall, but the *health which she is given*; a health that clashes with her desire of becoming-free. What eventually changes is not her awareness of what constitutes risky practice. It is her flow of desire that shifts, rendering freedom possible through her encounter with other assemblages. Situated in the recovery, rather than in the drug assem-blage at the time that this narrative becomes, the desire of becoming-other is enhanced through other encounters, where the substance is not present. Narratives like that, complicate the question of pleasure and freedom in a way that neoliberal and individualised understandings of health are unable to grasp. What is at stake here is not the maximisation of the pleasure that a substance can offer. Looking for 'better', 'healthier' or 'safer' ways of doing drugs does not appear to be relevant to the narrator's becoming with drugs. Conversely, in the narrator's drug assemblage, sex-work and living on the street are not discussed as negative consequences of her drug consumption, but as inextricable elements of her desired becoming-other, in this case, becoming-free, challenging 'the assumption that it must either be pleasure or pain that motivates risk-taking activities such as drug use' (Malins, 2017: 130). This way of thinking reflects Tuck's call for an epistemological shift from damage-centred research, to one that captures desire instead (2009). According to Tuck, 'desire-based research frameworks are connected with understanding complexity, contradiction, and the self-determination of lived lives ... by documenting not only the painful elements of social realities but also the wisdom and hope' (2009: 416). This epistemological shift does not install desire as an antonym to damage (ibid.: 419), but instead makes room for the contradictions (ibid.: 421) that traverse people's realities. The pain and suffering that very often comes with sex-work and homelessness is not sidelined but complicated, through the consideration of the flows of desire that it rendered possible at that specific time. Finally, once more, the substance is indirectly present and not in the focus of attention. Although sex-work is deployed as a means to acquire money for the purchase of drugs, the emphasis is on the capacity to *feel free* to do so while leaving an environment identified as oppressive at the time ('*I can't be home anymore, I can't stand this pressure*').

The accounts that follow though narrate another drug reality. Asking service-users if and how their relationship with drugs changed when drug use became a daily practice, the responses provided demonstrate a shift of the drug from an agent of becoming-other to an obstacle that blocks the flows of desire. The substance in these accounts is not just one element of the assemblage but the force that holds it together. Additionally, it is the force responsible for the service-users' lack of freedom. However, unlike the logic of systems of thought already criticised for not capturing the complexity and ambivalence of a body's becoming with drugs, this lack of freedom is not associated with 'wrong', 'unhealthy' choices but with the *lack of time* to become with other assemblages. While in the drug assemblages discussed until now the drug was mobilised to enhance the desired becomings, in the accounts that follow the substance dominates the service-users' lives, leaving no space or time for any other desire to flow:

> Yes [my relationship with drugs] did change because time was fractured. The time before using, the duration of use, the time after using where there would be conflict with the social, family, love environment because of the fact that I was using, so all this was violent and not relieving like at the beginning ... thinking about it now I'd say that while at the beginning I was using the substance as a fuel that could take me out in the world, 2-3 years later I couldn't be neither out there nor on my own without the influence of the substance.

In this account, drug use fractures time, decomposing the collective body's relations. The substance, used originally as a fuel to augment a body's capacity to act (*a fuel that could take me out in the world*) has shifted into an obstacle that blocks all lines of flight, external and internal.

> *The last 4 years I was using every 15 minutes. Using them both [heroin and cocaine] together, using one after a while to get the feeling I wanted, the balance, cause I didn't want the speed of coke, nor the gouching of the gear. I wanted the in-between ... I was looking for balance, but I never had that balance and I ended up using every 15 minutes.*

> *... until I got into it for good and I lived to use. I was waking up in the morning and my only concern was to find money, go to score, go to use, hang out a bit and then anything else.*

> *But then I'd wake up eventually and just start again, I was like I do not want to face another day. It was that, it was a constant battle of just facing the day. And my only way of dealing with it or trying to escape the day was to just do what I'd been doing, just carry on drinking, drink, drink, drink, and just try and block it all out.*

Up until now, the main common element of the narratives shared has been the desire of becoming-other, a desire where the substance is the agent but not the protagonist. In the above narratives the drug is not just the protagonist, but the *sole actor* of these stories of daily use, where there is no space or time left for any other desire to flow. In the first narrative, time is fractured and re-composed around the moments that precede and proceed the consumption of the substance. In the second one the desire of becoming-balanced is never accomplished, and yet drug use remains the force around which time is measured, while in the last two narratives any desire of becoming-other has been sidelined by time-consuming drug using routines. Simplifying the question of drug use and freedom, based on the empirical data produced, I argue that the drug user does not lack freedom because she fails to make healthy and responsible choices, but because any desire of becoming-other has been blocked and absorbed by a repetition of drug-using practices that keep blocking instead of releasing the flows of desire. Following Deleuze, these narratives are examples of 'bad' encounters, as 'the collective body is no longer propelled by its own desire, but focused on repelling, or expelling the "bad" encounter, such that all its force of existence is immobilised' (McLeod, 2017: 139). They are accounts of flows of desires that might have enabled transformation, but translated instead to an unease or fear that triggered passionate attempts at averting, preventing, controlling and blocking the flows (Malins, 2017: 128).

The way drug using time is organised also needs to be accounted for in relation to the socialities within which it becomes. Ethnographic and other empirical studies have demonstrated how social, economic and financial apparatuses lead to the stigmatisation and criminalisation of drug use and the entrapment of drug users in a vicious circle of practices that re-enforces their classification as solely drug using subjectivities (Bourgois, 1995). Kelly Knight (2015) has specifically addressed the issue of the multiple temporalities that traverse her participants' daily lives:

> In the daily-rent hotels the concrete routines of living called on women to meet unrelenting, and often conflicting, temporal demands. Ramona, like all the other addicted, pregnant women who resided in the daily-rent hotels, operated in multiple 'time zones' every day. She was on 'addict time', repeatedly searching for crack and heroin and satiating her addiction to them. 'Pregnancy time' reminded her that her expanding womb was a ticking time bomb. On 'hotel time' she constantly needed to hustle up her rent through daily sex work.
>
> (Knight, 2015: 8)

Accordingly, legal economies of drug use, like methadone maintenance programmes, have been critically explored for regulating and managing the temporalities of the dug using body, blocking its capacity to perform outside this identity (Bourgois, 2000; Fraser and valentine, 2008). Overall, whether discussing illicit drug use or substitution,

> Addiction can only be recognised by the presence of structure, patterns and rituals. A total collapse into uncontrolled and meaningless chaos would probably not be able to be interpreted at all, except possibly at psychosis. The parameters of control and rules of consumption followed by the addict may be regarded as negligible or indeed remain invisible to others, but this does not decrease their importance in regulating and structuring behaviour.
>
> (Keane, 2002: 58)

Focusing on the service-users' narratives, my aim has not been to account for all the social, political and economic components of the drug assemblage, but to follow the thread of the desire of becoming-other mediated by drug use, until the point where it becomes blocked. Through these empirical accounts it has been demonstrated that while '… productive desire can enable people to realise what *else* a body can do' (Fox, 2012: 111), the desire mediated by drug use eventually diminished a body's capacity to act. Instead of becoming 'something more, something else, someone freed from a sense of lacking an object or another person' (Fox, 2012: 110), the desire of becoming-other is blocked when the drug shifts from an agent, to an all time-consuming purpose. This is reflected on the shift of the position of the drug in the narratives of the service-users, from a component present but not the locomotive of desire, to the sole desired component of an assemblage.

Thinking with desire and time challenges the conceptualisation of addiction in opposition to pleasure (Dennis, 2019: 55), and brings to the forefront the potentiality of thinking drug use otherwise, in a way that does not position the substance, but the desired becomings in the focus of attention. Before moving on to the exploration of the recovery assemblage, where the affective relations that enable the flows of desire to become without the substance are produced, I return to Deleuze's turning point. Instead though of talking about the turning point associated with becoming a user, in what follows I focus on the turning points that lead towards the desire of becoming a service-user. Staying with the empirical accounts of people in recovery, becoming a service-user is discussed as a potentiality that evolves through the amalgam of practices of care that one experiences while using. Following this line of thought, my aim is once more to challenge the need for a policy-driven segregation between harm reduction and recovery practices.

Turning points – becoming a service-user

maybe it's someone that has not been hurt at all, maybe it's someone dying, and the people around us just keep moving. Maybe time has stopped, right in that moment. Maybe every second feels like a century and the passers-by just go on with their little lives, going to work, shopping.

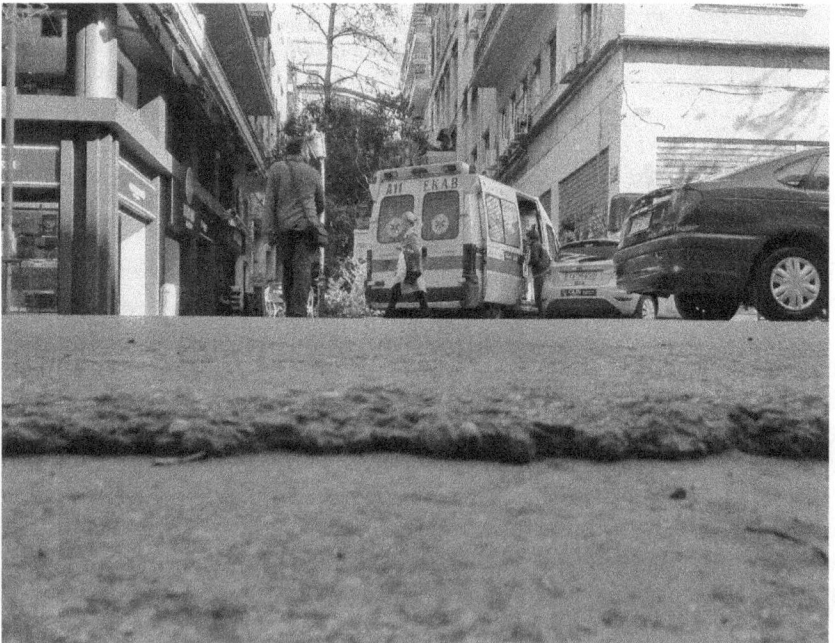

Figure 5.1 An ambulance in Athens.

In Figure 5.1, taken by one of the service-users during one of our photography walks, an ambulance is captured from a low angle, as if the photographer is the one lying on the street waiting to be picked up. His comment on it provides a different understanding of time and a closure to the previous ways that time was talked about: there is no acceleration of speed (Deleuze and Guattari, 2004), nor the potential of becoming slow and light, desired by some of the service-users; not even the repetitive temporality that blocked the desire of becoming-free. In this account time has stopped altogether.

In the first part of this chapter, the turning point was deployed to account for first experiences of drug use, the time that drug use *made sense* in a different way, addressing the service-users' desires of becoming. I now go back to the turning point to account for the participants' decisions to significantly alter their drug using practices or quit drugs. As the picture above indicates, moments in people's lives where time stops can be experienced as turning points, leading to life-changing decisions. Overdoses, diagnoses of drug-related illnesses, the death of another user, are often events narrated as fractures with time, 'rock-bottoms', turning points, associated with people's decisions to 'ask for help' (Kemp, 2013; Kirouac, Frohe and Witkiewitz, 2015; Shinebourne and Smith, 2010). In the data produced there are a series of narratives where 'hitting rock bottom', non-fatal overdoses or other life-altering, life-damaging or nearly life-interrupting experiences have informed the service-users' decisions to engage with recovery services. When following however their narratives on this decision, it became apparent that this was not solely informed by negative experiences, but also by positive encounters of care with people that had gone through recovery, as well as with harm reduction practitioners. The focus here is on those encounters, providing a first empirical approach on how practices of care, inside and beyond the recovery assemblage, matter.

As discussed earlier in this chapter, Deleuze (1990), draws on the writings of Fitzgerald (1945) and Lowry (1965) with alcohol, to account for a subjectivity's 'crack', the noisy accidents that happen inside and outside, leading to

> *a silent, imperceptible crack, at the surface, a unique surface Event ... the crack pursues its silent course, changes direction following the lines of least resistance, and extends its web only under the immediate influence of what happens, until sound and silence wed each other intimately and continuously in the shattering and bursting of the end. What this means is that the entire play of the crack has become incarnated in the depth of the body, at the same time that the labor of the inside and the outside has widened the edges.*
> (Deleuze, 1990: 155)

The question that Deleuze subsequently asks is how can we contain this silent trace of the incorporeal fact at the surface, how can we prevent the crack from deepening in the thickness of the noisy body? (ibid.: 156–157). I address this question by following how encounters of care between service-users and (a) people in recovery and (b) workers of harm reduction services, contained the crack by enhancing a new desire, that of becoming a service-user:

> *The first fellowship I got involved in was [name of the service], came by chance really, it was an old school friend of mine who's part of the team there, and we'd lost touch for many years and it was just by chance I bumped into him one day at Lime Street Station, and he could see I was in a bad way at the time and he asked how I was and I told him everything and he just, he just suggested about like the [name of the service], if I'd be interested in engaging, taking part, and I said I absolutely would, yeah, because I mean for twenty two years I'd been looking for help, but I wasn't finding anything that suited me, I was going to see my GP, regularly and I was basically pleading for help because I needed it, and all I was getting told was to go to the Royal and speak to the crisis team, which I'd done so many times but absolutely nothing [came] from it. So meeting up with my old mate from school and getting involved in the [name of the service], that gave me a start.*

> *I went to the hospital to have two abscesses cleaned and as I came out I saw this guy that I used to use [drugs] with, and he was always a mess and staying on the streets. And I suddenly saw him and he was fine! He said he had been clean for 6-7 years, working in the hospital and had two kids. And I'm like, where the fuck did you go and what did you do? And he said 'here, just across the street [where one of the services of 18 ano is], you should go'. And I instantly thought if he did it, I can do it too! Not to underestimate him, I just didn't expect it.*

While shared drug-using practices and solidarity among drug users have been explored as ways to minimise harm, as well as to create bonds of intimacy and care (Bourgois and Schonberg, 2009; Farrugia, 2015; Fraser et al., 2014; Manton et al., 2014), little attention has been paid to the interactions between people in recovery and active users. The narratives above account for two such interactions. By both service-users they are described as unplanned meetings with people from their past, producing turning points that led to their engagement with services. The first encounter is described as an unexpected offer for care, provided by an 'old mate', rather than by the institutions expected to take that role (*'I was going to see my GP, regularly and I was basically pleading for help because I needed it, and all I was getting told was to go to the Royal and speak to the crisis team, which I'd done so many times but absolutely nothing [came] from it'*). According to the service-user, it was this unexpected encounter that 'gave him a start'. The second narrative accounts for an equally unexpected encounter, leading to the narrator's engagement with

18 ano. Following the meeting with a former drug using acquaintance, a new option becomes available: *if he did it, I can do it too!* This sudden realisation of the existence of other possibilities appears to activate a hidden, or not previously known desire, the desire of becoming without drugs. In the accounts above, turning points are not talked about as 'rock bottom' experiences of use, but as unexpected encounters with people outside the drug assemblage, encounters that enhance one's life possibilities and activate the desire to connect with other assemblages.

Staying with the intention to challenge the assumption that harm reduction and recovery address different and conflicting desires, the following empirical narratives talk about harm reduction as a practice of care that stays with the crack but prevents it from deepening irremediably (Deleuze, 1990: 157). By 'being there' and caring for drug users, harm reduction practitioners enhance the production of affective relations that allow for the possibility of recovery to remain open. Unlike the encounters discussed above, the experiences that follow account for the turning point as it becomes through a process, through consistent encounters rather than unexpected ones:

> *You know what, I was feeling really nice when I was seeing them. There was this instant sense of warmth … They were trying to encourage me to stop using and become something like a coordinator [for the service]. They wanted me to. They were seeing something in me. I never made it but … I think they had an influence on me. Seeing people standing on their feet, addressing the difficulties without becoming one with them, and they just ask you to try and they treat you like nobody has treated you before. Because in society drug users are not treated well. Having people to take care for you even at your worst for me is very important. It was also through them that I learned about 18 [ano], I can't remember exactly when but it stayed in my mind, and years later I called [at 18 ano].*

> *Just the fact that some people who aren't using come there and care for me being on the street made me feel well. I was also a bit ashamed but I was feeling well.*

Reflecting the experiences discussed earlier, the service-users above account for the possibilities opened up through connections with other assemblages. This time the encounters are not unexpected but consistent. What appears to matter for the narrators is the presence of non-users in a drug using environment, the fact that the harm reduction practitioners chose to become part of the drug assemblage, in order to care for those within it. While the presence of the drug-user in the environments of use is talked about as a necessity, the engagement of non-users with the using space is talked about as a choice, expanding the life possibilities of those who feel unable to extend to other assemblages. The practitioners' differentiation from the drug assemblage is of equal importance ('*Seeing people standing on their feet, addressing the difficulties without becoming one with them …*', '*Just the fact that some people who aren't using come there and care for me being on the street made me feel well*'). Paraphrasing Deleuze, what appears to matter for the narrators is the encounters and connections with people that were there to see for themselves, to be a little alcoholic, a little crazy, a little suicidal, to stay at the surface without staying on the shore (Deleuze, 1990: 157–158). Turning points in that sense are the outcomes of connections whose meaningfulness gradually evolves, expanding life possibilities. These connections are not produced over big gestures and radical changes, but primarily through the provision of caring practices that aim to ameliorate the lives of people within the environments they inhabit:

> *There was this van coming to take care of you, to give you food … there was also a space where you could have a shower, have a coffee, get condoms … I was so happy when the food was coming and we were eating all together, sometimes I was crying. I was getting emotional.*

In this narrative, it is a daily practice experienced in a collective way that activates one's emotions. Addressing drug users' needs in situ does more than meeting these immediate needs. It demonstrates in practice how these daily encounters can be experienced differently. In the account that follows the same issues are addressed from the perspective of a worker at a residential service for young people:

> *I remember there was this girl using crack, pills, heroin, cocaine, skunk, anything you can think of. What she needed was someone to take care of her, to prepare some food … It was so exhausting what she was going through that recovery couldn't be the first approach. You just need to be there for her, make her breakfast, take her for a walk, take her to the doctor. Be there and remind them bit by bit that they are humans, because they live under very difficult and risky situations, especially the girls.*

The aim of the worker here is to facilitate a young woman's daily life *and* to actively work out with her a way for life to be done differently; to navigate with her potential turning points that can activate hidden flows of desire.

The turning point from becoming a user to becoming a service-user might happen unexpectedly, through unplanned encounters, as discussed through the first narratives. It might also be something to work on collectively by the drug-users and those that care for them, understood as a process, an amalgam of small gestures of care that address direct needs while simultaneously opening up new life possibilities. These are all practices aiming at maintaining the crack in the surface, preventing it from entering deeper and rooting in one's body. This containment of the crack on the surface is not subject to general rules (Deleuze, 1990: 160). Practices of harm reduction and recovery are entangled, consistently and patiently working towards the enhancement of the connections between bodies and the production of affective practices that lead to turning points, whether these take place within the territoriality of the drug or the recovery assemblage. Finally, it is important to emphasise that the 'cracks' shared since the beginning of this chapter, are not parentheses of people's lives, breaks between wellbeing. They are intrinsic components of the service-users' narratives of becoming-well (McLeod, 2017). The desires flowing through substances are not accounts of loss and despair, but of hope. Desire is involved with the *not yet*, as much as it is with the *not anymore* (Tuck, 2009: 417, emphasis in original). Accounts of becoming-blocked through drugs were expressions of the *not yet*. The chapter that follows explores the material, affective and social assemblages of recovery that become when desire gets involved with the *not anymore*.

Notes

1 All italicised quotes are from my interviews with service-users, unless stated otherwise.
2 Vathis square, Pedio to Areos and Menidi are Athenian areas known for drug dealing and drug using activities.

Chapter 6

The recovery assemblage

The previous chapter followed the investment of the service-users' desire through substances, and accounted for the turning points that shifted this desire. Experiences of drug use that *made sense*, eventually led to the domination of all the assemblages that the using body was extending to by the substance, blocking becomings and flows of desire. Therefore, another turning point came into being, addressing the shifting desire of becoming a drug user to becoming a service-user. The connections that rendered this shift possible were produced by consistent and unexpected encounters of care, offering hints of how desire can potentially flow without the substances. In what follows I am staying with desire and care to explore the connections produced when that last turning point materialises and one becomes a service-user through their engagement with the recovery assemblage.

> *[Deleuze and Guattari] teach us that desire is assembled, crafted over a lifetime through our experiences. For them, this assemblage is the picking up of distinct bits and pieces that, without losing their specificity, become integrated into a dynamic whole. This is what accounts for the multiplicity, complexity and contradiction of desire, how desire reaches for contrasting realities, even simultaneously … Exponentially generative, engaged, engorged, desire is not mere wanting but our informed seeking.*
>
> (Tuck, 2009: 418)

In this chapter the recovery assemblage is unpacked as a collective effort to pick up bits and pieces, destratified desires and hopes for the future, and to integrate them into a dynamic whole. The multiplicity and contradiction of desire is not 'resolved' but allowed to unfold in all its complexity and to flow through the affective and caring relations produced. This chapter brings together Duff's methodology for the exploration of the assemblage in recovery from mental illness with the empirical accounts of people in recovery. Duff (2014a) identifies three assemblages of health that enable the emergence of recovery from mental illness: the social, material and affective assemblage.

DOI: 10.4324/9781003165613-7

The focus initially is on the material assemblage of recovery, to account for the discrete territories of the assemblage, as well as for their purposes, meanings and functions (Duff, 2014a: 103–104). I then move on to the affective assemblage to investigate how the caring practices produced in the recovery space enhance a body's capacity to act. Finally, the social assemblage is discussed as a collective formation of connections becoming within the recovery assemblage and extending beyond it, thus rendering deterritorialisations possible. Although the material, affective and social aspects of the recovery assemblage are simultaneously constitutive of all its practices, by focusing on each one of them separately renders all these forces visible through specific empirical examples. Closely attending to the forces that traverse the recovery assemblage, I account for the composition and assemblage of health 'from among the affects, signs, forces and events that inflect a body's power of acting' (Duff, 2014a: 118).

Care is an affective and selective mode of attention to some things and not to others (Martin, Myers and Viseau, 2015), and by unpacking the material, affective and social assemblages of recovery, the aim is to challenge the constitution of the recovery practice as one solely caring for the interruption of the relationship between a body and a substance. Shifting the attention from the interruption to the enhancement of connections and socialities, I attend to the service-users' desire of becoming without drugs. In the introduction to this book, it was emphasised that this is not an attempt to provide generalising assumptions and guidelines about how recovery should be done. The analysis that follows reflects the practices, encounters and connections becoming in two specific recovery assemblages, and the experiences of the service-users and workers producing those assemblages at a specific time.

The material recovery assemblage

While Duff's (2014a) focus is on the ways that social inclusion and community participation enhance the body's becoming-well from mental illness, my exploration of the material and affective assemblage of recovery addresses the connections produced *within* the territory of recovery, and how these connections 'affect transitions and becomings arising in subsequent encounters within subsequent assemblages' (Andrews and Duff, 2019: 125). This does not mean that the recovery space becomes in isolation. Its relationship to the 'outside', its constitution as penetrable and yet other to what lies beyond its territory is essential for the understanding of the affective connections that become possible within the recovery space. To account for this relationship, I return to Foucault's (1986) analysis of heterotopias, to explore how the production of the services' present territories render them 'other spaces', reflections of the societies within which they emerge and they speak about and yet absolutely different from them (Foucault, 1986: 25).

I will initially focus on the participants' first encounters with the recovery services, as spaces that 'presuppose a system of opening and closing that both isolates them and makes them penetrable' (Foucault, 1986: 28). I discuss the production of the material recovery assemblage, specifically looking at how its territoriality is unfolded through the process of 'turning up' for an assessment appointment, and how the recovery space is extended beyond its physical territory through the process of 'checking in' with the service-users when they are not physically present at the recovery space.

Turning-up and assessment appointments

During the time that I was working at the reception of Genie, there were several occasions when people walked in to ask information about the service, see the space and express their interest in engaging with recovery. Although these queries were always treated in a welcoming way, passers-by were never allowed to spend a lot of time in the reception, walk into groups and, in general, interact with the service-users. Their interest was usually addressed by any member of staff available at the area of the reception or in an office if the conversation had to be private, and the visitor would be accompanied to the door once the visit had come to an end. The responsibility of the worker on-site is to offer all guests the information on the 'admission process', including, using Foucault's terms, the gestures that have to be made, the rites and purifications that the newcomer has to be submitted to in order to get permission to access the space as a service-user (Foucault, 1986: 28), while ensuring the physical and symbolic segregation between the 'outsiders' and the recovery space. It is at this very initial stage, the first contact with the service, that the territoriality and the affective relationships that define the recovery assemblage start taking shape.

The first step towards 'becoming a service-user' is to make an appointment and turn up for an assessment. This is a practical – as a member of staff qualified to conduct the assessment must be available at the time – but most importantly a symbolic gesture, a commitment from both sides that on a chosen day they will make time for each other. It is this commitment that becomes the first point of negotiation between the potential service-user and the service, and it requires patience and work from all actors involved. It is the agreement to 'share time' with each other that initiates the production of both the territoriality as well as the temporality of the recovery assemblage. Drug use time though is a non-linear, complicated experience that very often clashes with normative understandings of time, including the ability to keep appointments (Fraser and valentine, 2008; Knight, 2015). In my experience from Genie, assessment appointments would very often not show up, in most cases without cancelling in advance. It then becomes the responsibility of the worker to contact the person that missed their appointment, ask them if they are well and invite them to book another one. This 'ritual of admission' can be a lengthy and time-consuming process, occasionally successful, occasionally not, but in any case, a first attempt to establish a committed and caring relationship. Therefore, the assessment appointment stands symbolically as a threshold (Latimer, 2018: 380) that potential service-users must pass, accompanied by service-workers, in order to become part of the recovery assemblage. Passing this threshold is an active affirmation of the service-user's desire for care and a service-worker's commitment to provide this care.

These difficulties and the importance of the first contact resonates with 18 ano's head of research experience:

> *We statistically know that out of 100 addicts that are going to call, only 60 will show up for their appointment at least once, and then you give a fight to keep them [coming back]. The first appointment is very important and a very difficult job. You have to do your best, in your own way, your sensitivity, your knowledge, your experience, to say something that's going to make sense and will make them come back. And the percentage of those that keep coming back after two months is 20% and the aim is to make it 21%.*

By asking the potential service-user to attend an appointment, drug use time clashes with recovery time; the time and space of the user is disrupted. '[Recovery] heterotopias draw [the users] out of [them]selves in peculiar ways; they display and inaugurate a difference and challenge the space in which [they] may feel at home' (Johnson, 2006: 84). The importance of managing to 'turn up' for this first appointment is highlighted in the following account through the frustration caused when this achievement is not properly acknowledged:

> *I booked an appointment, and they told me come on the 12th of the month, I can't really remember the exact date, at 10am, and I was there at 10am sharp, something that hardly ever happens and they told me I wasn't on the list! Although I'd made a note of it and everything! I was fuming, I left and I was like fuck that! I got on my bike and when I had almost reached Omonia square [to score drugs] they called me and they're like, we're so sorry, there has been a mistake, could you please come back? And I thought about it ... and went back for the appointment, and the second and the third one ... [Name of the key-worker] helped me a lot because I understood that I could trust her. She was listening what I was telling her and believing it and I could see that she saw something in me. And that's how I started [the recovery process].*

The narrative above begins with the expression of anger caused when 'turning up' is not acknowledged. This highlights the significance of the decision to 'turn up' at the recovery space, as a shift of the desired becomings. When this desire is blocked by the recovery space, the immediate response of the narrator is to return to his familiar 'using' space, until an apologetic phone call disrupts his decision, and makes him 'think about it'. As his relationship with his key worker evolves his distance from the drug using space and time keeps growing. The otherness of the recovery space 'is established through a relationship of difference with other sites, such that their presence either provides an unsettling of spatial and social relations or an alternative representation of spatial and social relations' (Hetherington, 1997: 8).

Checking-in, ticking boxes and birthday cards

Neoliberal systems of thought present the drug user as a 'free' subject that can make informed, 'healthy' choices and respectively take responsibility for those choices and actions. The reality however of the initial encounter between the service and the user, reveals the process of 'asking for help' as a non-linear, complex one, where the practices of care are not known in advance:

> *I didn't know [what to expect] to be honest. I just wanted to go and see. I wanted to see what's this help that they say that they give you.*

Through this statement the desire to understand and connect with the material assemblage of recovery is expressed. Through this connection recovery shifts from an abstract formation into a specific practice taking place at a space where one has to physically *go* in order to *see* what kind of help can be given. Exploring the process and practices of 'asking for help' in all their complexity and heterogeneity serves to challenge the neoliberal production of subjectivity through which responsibility is placed on the individual and its ability to make informed 'healthy' choices. Annemarie Mol (2008) argues that the 'logic of choice' dominates healthcare, and she proposes instead a 'logic of care' where the needs of each subject are navigated collectively by the user, the worker and the service. The provision of care becomes thus a shared responsibility, a co-participation that requires all actors (non-human and human) involved to shift their practices in order to engage with each other in ways that unblock the desired becomings and enhance a body's capacity to act.

An example of an approach to care in the recovery assemblage that challenges the 'logic of choice' is Genie's daily practice of 'checking-in' with the service-users by calling them. One of the daily tasks of workers at Genie is to send a text (SMS) to all the service-users that details Genie's activities for the day. The workers then call as many service-users as possible, first thing in the morning, to ask how they are doing and encourage them to 'come in' for the day. This is a task that requires attention to and knowledge of each service-user's schedule. For example, during my fieldwork at Genie, being there on Mondays and Tuesdays, after a while I knew which service-users were expected to show up, and which ones would not due to other commitments. It was my responsibility every Monday and Tuesday morning to call the 'regular' service-users of those days, and those that had not shown up for a while and check-in with them. This practice extends beyond the physical territory of the recovery assemblage, reaching out to other assemblages that the service-users operate within. By caring for them, whether they are physically present at the recovery space or not, the recovery assemblage is extended beyond a specific territoriality. This small gesture was very often commented upon during the interviews with service-users as being important for them as a practice of care that increased their engagement with the service:

> *yeah, with Genie, they do care about the clients and they do keep an eye on you, they send you texts and they phone you up.*

> *I did come along and after a while I stopped coming along, I thought I didn't need to and I was drinking for quite a while ... and [member of staff] she called me one day and asked me to come back and I did and I've been coming back since.*

The service-users value Genie's practice of 'checking-in' as a consistent attempt to establish a stable attachment and connection between the service-user and the service. The fact that the workers 'keep an eye on you' is experienced as a caring practice, potentially leading to turning points for the reconnection with the service in cases when the process of becoming a service-user has been interrupted (*I stopped coming along ... she called me one day and ... I've been coming back since*). Within a logic of choice, this practice could be evaluated as time-consuming, unnecessary and even harmful in that it could undermine the service-users' agency. Considering that the service-user has already been given information regarding the schedule of the service, the practice of calling non-attenders could be seen as undermining their choice to not show up. Furthermore, sidelining the specifics of their daily lives, it could be framed as non-compliance with the service's requirements and lack of desire to establish meaningful connections. However, service-users' narratives tell a different story that enacts the practice of 'checking-in' as care and in turn complicates the question of agency and emphasises the ambivalences that inform their daily decisions:

> *they're very nice people here and you know quite friendly bunch and non-judgemental and supportive and, they give you a kick up the arse if you need the motivation, and they can tell if you, you're down and they try to bring you up again and get you moved back up and I, I realise that this time they meant it! They were actually trying to help and they are nice people and they are doing it for the right reasons, whereas before I kind of got the impression that they were just trying to tick boxes and say, and show willing, you know ... So usually, because I'm quite intelligent, perceptive, so I can tell*

the difference between people who mean it and people who don't mean it. So I think I, you know I suppose I felt sort of welcomed here more genuinely than I did like say when I went on the CBT course because that was more a case of just someone whose job it is to do this for a couple of weeks with this patient, you know to, you know show that the NHS is doing something, to show that, I don't know some politician set that up at some point, did something, whatever!

In the accounts above, making choices is talked about as a process that requires '*a kick up the arse if you need the motivation*', as well as the occasional phone call from a worker that asks the service-user to come back and re-engage with the service. These narratives challenge the constitution of service-users as autonomous individuals that make personal choices, disassociated from their encounters with others. Conversely, 'making choices' is talked about as a situated and relational process where the encounters with others matter, and the affective relations in place have the power to change the course of this process. In other words, 'making choices' in the recovery assemblage is not about making the 'right' choice following a linear path that leads to abstinence, but about experiencing the caring practices that render the desired becoming-other possible.

The processes of 'turning up' and 'checking in' are caring practices of the material recovery assemblage, producing a territoriality that takes into consideration the everyday realities of service-users. The narrative above emphasises another component of the material assemblage that very often dominates drug services: the process of 'ticking boxes' and filling out forms. In the quote that follows, the manager of Genie talks about these forms as meaningful components of the material assemblage of recovery only when they contribute to the establishment of affective connections:

[It's not about] getting someone in and filling out the form, well I've filled out that form so you go home, have a good weekend. It's about making sure it's a reality, you know. Is that form, is that going to help this person to get through the weekend? Are they going to walk out of here and they've got somewhere to go, you know?

'Turning up' for an assessment appointment is a collective effort that takes into consideration the everyday realities of service-users. Staying with this commitment, 'checking in' stabilises this relationship of care. Accordingly, 'filling out forms' matters when it works towards the establishment of the connections and support required, when it leads to the provision of this support in practice rather than in paper, '*making sure it's a reality*'. Finally, another practice of Genie, deployed to enhance the connection between the service and its users – whether their presence is consistent or not – is the posting of birthday cards:

A lot of people come and they, you know, they get a birthday card from us,
it's not rocket science, but a lot of them don't have anyone. And that makes
someone come back we've not seen in months, you saw [name of service-
user] before, we haven't seen him about a year, but he would have got a
birthday card from us.

Through this practice the presence of the service remains consistent even
when the presence of the service-user in the recovery service is not. Through
the birthday card, the material recovery assemblage extends beyond a specific
territoriality and reaches out to the service-users' personal spaces. The fact
that none of the service-users ever gets crossed off the birthday list, no matter
for how long they had not 'turned up' at the service, constitutes a resistance to
recovery models that follow a logic of choice that 'punishes' the service-users'
occasional inconsistency by interrupting their connection with the service.

Tracing these material practices as they become within the recovery assemblage leads to an understanding of the practices of care unfolding in the
recovery space that goes beyond their measurability or potential translata-
bility into policy documents. The 'success' of mental health interventions
like CBT courses is usually measured through feedback forms that enable the
quantification of participants' responses. However, non-quantifiable elements, like the connection between these practices and the daily realities of
service-users are systematically sidelined by these short-term approaches of
recovery. Conversely, what the empirical testimonies of the service-users have
emphasised is the importance of gestures that establish the service and its
users as co-authors of the recovery process; practices that create a shared
responsibility by generating the feeling that '*[the workers of a service] do care*
about [them]', that '*[they] keep an eye on [them]*', and '*can tell if you're*
down'. These accounts indicate *how* care matters and, more specifically, how
unmeasurable practices of care matter.

Following this line of thought, looks at the service-users' agency through a
new prism: it shifts the focus of attention from the provision of information
that will lead to 'healthy', informed decisions, to the deployment of caring
practices that create a shared commitment between the user and the service.
Through their accounts it becomes obvious that not only can they '*tell the*
difference between people who mean it and people who don't mean it', but also
that they *care* about whether they mean it or not, they can tell when the provision of 'care' reflects an attempt to '*tick boxes*'. Through these narratives a
'desire for care' is articulated, a desire for meaningful, affective relationships
that become through unmeasurable caring practices.

Becoming safe

As we gradually shift from the exploration of the material to the affective
recovery assemblage, I focus on how the practices discussed above produce the

recovery space as 'safe'. This safety refers to the territoriality of the recovery, as well as to the connections enhanced through the specific ways in which recovery is practised, making the affective assemblage possible. According to Foucault, the heterotopia's role 'is to create a space that is other, another real space, as perfect, as meticulous, as well arranged as ours is messy, ill constructed, and jumbled' (Foucault, 1986: 29). However, the recovery space is not perfect and meticulous. On the contrary, conflict, doubt and negotiation are integral elements of the recovery assemblage and the affective flows that define it. Through the exploration of the therapeutic relationship and the feeling of 'safety', the otherness of the recovery space and the lines of flight that this other space opens, come into shape:

> It's the safest place I've ever known. Honestly, that's how I experienced it. There were times that I was coming back here cos I couldn't stand being out there ... By safe I mean that I was feeling calm ... (drug) use can't reach you.

> The people are lovely and the staff are really great. It's just I feel safe here. It's somewhere I can get out and do something, get out of the hostel ... it's that atmosphere, the arguing, the money, the arguing about drugs, and that's not for me, I don't want to be in that situation. I'd rather get out and do something.

> I've never had the advantage before of having a space clean, safe, with a safety net that no matter how hard I fall will hold me and I'll stand up, and lots of love and understanding with everything.

The recovery space is talked about in juxtaposition to the 'outside' ('I was coming back here cos I couldn't be out there'), as the place to go to in order to leave another environment ('It's somewhere I can get out and do something, get out of the hostel'), and as a space where falling becomes possible (a space clean, safe, with a safety net that no matter how hard I fall will hold me'). In all three accounts, safety is the primary feeling that leads the participants to stay in or return to the recovery space. Safety is associated with feeling calm and the existence of protective mechanisms. It is also linked to the lack of substances and other drug using activities ('drug use can't reach you'). Finally, and as explained by the keyworker of Genie, the aim of the service is to render the recovery space 'more attractive' than the 'using space':

> In the end my belief is coming back here becomes more attractive than going back there and I don't know how long that process takes.

The narratives of workers regarding their relationship with service-users show that for the recovering space to become safe and attractive, the absence of substances is not enough. An 'alternate ordering' (Hetherington, 1997: 9) has to be in place, which will allow new conditions of sociality to come into being' (ibid: 17), as discussed by Genie's key worker:

> *I see these guys that are amazingly skilful in some areas of their life and it's been neglected and put down and left to go dusty in the corner and on the other side of that, the part the world sees is this dysfunctional, unmanageable person and that's not the person, that's the person in that kind of situation. We see them in all regards. We see the real person, the ups, the downs, the this, the that, and we don't offer them solutions. You're just offering them a space really, say it's okay, you can feel safe in here, you can be yourself in here and then we gradually watch them become themselves.*

As Johnson notes, a major problem with Foucault's account of heterotopias 'concerns the question of the extent of their "difference" and how such difference can be measured' (Johnson, 2013: 793). Based on the account above, there is a 'difference' between what '*the world sees*' and what the recovery workers see. The provision of a safe space is how this 'difference' comes into being, a space where people, by being themselves eventually also *become* themselves. The service-users' accounts demonstrate that it is not simply the provision of a space that creates safety, but the affective relationships produced within the recovery assemblage that render becoming-other possible. The recovery setting does not just provide space for difference; the heterotopia of recovery '*makes* differences and unsettles spaces' (Johnson, 2013: 796, emphasis in original). This difference is not made by the replacement of the 'outside' norms with new ones, but through alternate 'orderings' where relationships and connections are positioned in the focus of attention, as stated below by one of the therapists of 18 ano:

> *What I'm trying to do isn't to put them in norms that they would necessarily have to follow, apart from the basic principles and boundaries [of the programme]. What I'm trying to do as a therapist is manage to understand them and listen to them. So, I believe that that's what they really need, [the therapist] to build a good relationship with them, a corrective relationship let's say but with their own participation.*

When exploring the desire of becoming-other through the accounts of people in recovery, it was argued that although the substance was part of the becoming-other assemblage, it was not the only, nor the primary actor. Accordingly, in the therapeutic encounter it is not the substance positioned in the focus of attention, but the 'corrective' relationship built within the recovery assemblage. The foundation of the therapeutic relationship is not the establishment of norms that everyone must embrace, but the exploration of the desire of becoming-other and how it can flow instead of becoming blocked. What the therapeutic relationship comes to 'correct' is not the person, but the components of the assemblage that eventually blocked the flow of desire. Following Deleuze and Guattari's ambivalences, it has been discussed how desire, as much as it can enhance affective relations, 'also has the power to produce images that enslave it' (Colebrook, 2001: 94). The 'difference' that the heterotopia of recovery makes is the allowance for 'new conditions of sociality to come into being' (Hetherington, 1997: 9), a 'corrective' sociality that traces the flow of desire, the point where it became blocked. Hence the ongoing juxtaposition between the 'outside' and the recovery space is present in both recovery assemblages explored here. 'Heterotopias are not separate from society; they are distinct *emplacements*, that are "embedded" in all cultures and mirror, distort and react to the remaining space' (Johnson, 2013: 794, emphasis in original). The recovery assemblage does not stand in isolation, but in conflict, negotiation and in accordance with the society within which it evolves, where those excluded are 'seen' and 'heard', where norms are not imposed but under negotiation, where new, 'corrective' relations become possible. 'These connections and productions eventually form social wholes; when bodies connect with other bodies to enhance their power they eventually form communities or societies' (Colebrook, 2001: 91):

> In general, I couldn't have imagined that I'd have to radically change my everyday life, enter a residential stage that lasts for seven months where I wouldn't have any contact with my family or social circle, I, who used to talk to my parents on the phone ten times per day at least! I suddenly entered a house, the residential stage, where all contact was violently interrupted. There was a rupture in time and it was just me and myself ... There was a network of services and people and I was sharing everything with them, not with my mom, like I did in the past. I could talk with my personal or group therapist about everything. From the type of music that I like to a heartbreak that I had when I was fourteen and how that shaped me ... The relationship I had with the people around me was difficult and confrontational but I believe that without these people, [without] seeing them, living with them, building relationships with them on a daily basis, I wouldn't have managed to stay clean. With the world as it is outside I wouldn't have made it. In here people are clean.

The account above provides a link with McLeod's (2017) understanding of 'wellbeing', not as a linear 'success' story, but as an assemblage that takes illbeing seriously. The introduction of the service-user to the residential phase of recovery is described as a *'radical change'* of his everyday life, *'violently'* disrupting his time and space, reflecting the ways that heterotopias unsettle known spaces, draw subjectivities out of themselves and *make* differences. The juxtaposition between the 'inside' and the 'outside' is again present: *'with*

the world as it is outside I wouldn't have made it. In here people are clean'.
The word 'clean' refers to more than abstinence from substances; it reflects
the relationships built within the service, described as difficult and confrontational, and yet rendering a certain form of 'purification' possible, when
compared and contrasted to the world outside the recovery space. The network of services, the therapists, the other service-users, the daily contact
and conviviality with all these people are described as 'emplacements' of
relationships that were identified as problematic, destratifying flows of desire
and blocking the body's capacity to act. The description of this network
as 'corrective' refers to its production not in isolation, but as a response to
illbeing. The recovery space becomes a 'different' space, where another 'sociality' is possible, through the slow and attentive construction of difficult and
'corrective' relationships.

The focus until now has been on the components of the material recovery
assemblage. The process of becoming a service-user demands a shift from
'using' to 'recovery' time, disrupting the service-users' space and time, drawing
them out of themselves in unexpected ways. 'Turning up' for an assessment
can be complicated and in conflict with the novel service-user's daily practices.
This conflict is negotiated collectively, by the service-user and the service,
leading to the establishment of the territoriality of recovery, and the production of an affective relationship between the service-user and the workers.
'Checking-in' is a caring practice that extends beyond the space of recovery and
takes into consideration the complexity of service-users' lives. Such recovery
approaches are enactments of Mol's (2008) call for a shift from a logic of
choice to a logic of care, and subsequently steps towards the understanding
of recovery as a collective practice. The non-human material components of
the recovery assemblage, like text messages, assessment forms and birthday
cards, are also mobilised for the production of affective practices that respond
to the service-users' daily realities and need for support inside and beyond the
recovery assemblage. These experiences of care produce the recovery space as
safe. Having ensured safety, difficulties and the acknowledgement of conflict
are not a threat, but a way to unblock the desire of becoming-other, a way for
service-users to 'become themselves', as put by Genie's keyworker. Following
the accounts of the service-users and paying attention to their experiences of
becoming blocked, alternate orderings are produced, allowing the flows of
desire to re-emerge. In what follows, the emphasis shifts from the material to
the affective components of the assemblage, specifically focusing on the establishment of boundaries and the generation of hope.

The affective recovery assemblage

Affect is the force that constitutes the body's capacity to affect and be affected
by the world of bodies and things that it encounters (Duff, 2014a: 106).
According to Massumi, every time a body affects and is affected, a transition

has been made, a threshold has been passed (Massumi, 2002: 212). The affective recovery assemblage accounts for a body's trajectory, as it crosses thresholds. The material assemblage was discussed as the production of a safe, 'other' space, where the becoming-blocked body can recover its flows of desire. This process rendered the affective assemblage possible, where the demolition of the barriers that blocked the flow of desire is actualised.

Establishing boundaries

'Boundary' is a widely used term within recovery assemblages. It usually refers to the rules set to ensure the safety of service-users and workers, and the smooth daily operation of the recovery service. Common boundaries within a recovery assemblage are the restrictions on the relationships between the service-users (usually communication outside the service is discouraged, as well as any form of sexual/intimate relationship), and the possession of substances when present in the service. My focus here is on specific boundaries as these are defined and applied by 18 ano. As is the case with most recovery services, there are some 'fundamental' boundaries, that if breached result in the – usually temporary – exclusion of the service-user.[1] However, the ones I will be focusing on are the daily boundaries that accompany all aspects of life in the residential stage of the programme. These have to do with the daily operation of the house that the service-users share, the needs of the residents and the relationships among them. Examples of such boundaries are the rituals that accompany cooking and eating, the regulated use of shared products in the house, and the responsibility of all service-users to make sure that no resident feels isolated. These are all boundaries related to everyday practices, the way service-users organise their everyday lives and the provision of care to them and from them to the other members of the service. Following empirical narratives, my aim is to explore how these everyday boundaries, as they are set, negotiated and exercised in the residential stage of the programme, are experienced as practices of care that lead to alternate orderings where the desire of becoming-other is collectively explored.

Unlike those described as 'fundamental' boundaries, the ones addressed here are not unconditionally imposed, but constantly under negotiation and discussion. There is a discursive element that accompanies these everyday boundaries, one that contributes simultaneously to the differentiation of each individual, as well as to the affective flows that render conviviality an intrinsic part of the recovery process.

> *I'm more into self-discipline. I have to make something mine. Otherwise I can't defend it and support it. It's all about comprehension. For some reason it works. I also released my anger and it was good ... [while in the residential stage of the programme] when something made me angry*

I would say it but I also understood, there was a voice in my head telling me wait to see why it happens.

This is an account of a service-user's relationship to these everyday boundaries. Ownership as well as comprehension of the rules that accompany her everyday practices are presented as the reasons why she was prepared to accept them. Conflict is also present in this process. Anger is discussed as a feeling that finds its own place in the recovery assemblage, accepted, negotiated and treated without leading to destratifications that could jeopardise the stability of the recovery space. Following this discursive practice, the boundaries negotiated in the recovery assemblage have 'nothing to do with a limitation, ban, or imperative that would come from the outside' (Stengers, 2010: 42). They are constraints 'on the order of "holding together with others' (ibid: 43), on the cultivation of an ethics of care that connects the personal to the collective through an everyday doing (de la Bellacasa, 2010). According to the therapeutic principles of 18 ano, 'holding together with others' does not happen through the suppression of one's feelings of discomfort, but through the production of spaces where anger and conflict are not avoided as potentially disruptive, but encouraged to flow:

My therapists were telling me that it was like I didn't exist. In order to avoid conflict [I kept saying] that it's all fine, all good, and they were telling me it's not possible that nothing bothers you. But all these years that's what I'd been used to, to 'swallow' everything that bothered me. I was finding it really difficult to understand what was bothering me or to hold a position, [it was] like I didn't have an opinion at all. I was afraid to confront anyone.

In the narrative above one's affirmation of existence is identified with her ability to engage with conflict, challenge boundaries and confront others. Within this line of thought, the affective meaning of boundaries is not the production of a harmonious and non-conflictive coexistence, but the acknowledgement of each body's needs and desires, collectively negotiated. Boundaries are not put in place to solely constrain, but also to be challenged, to facilitate the rise of oppressed feelings and desires. This is reflected in the weekly discussions between 18 ano's members of staff. Service-users that comply with all aspects of the residential stage and avoid the expression of anger or the engagement with conflict are problematised, and the focus of the treatment team shifts towards the attempt to identify the forces that block these affective arrays of feelings from arising. This practice of the treatment team of 18 ano comes to demonstrate that everyday boundaries are not in place to prevent action but to enhance it. Those caring for the service-users in the recovery assemblage are not solely interested in the ability to respect boundaries but also in the ability to breach them, to challenge their necessity and renegotiate them collectively.

In the chapter 'Becoming a drug user – becoming a service-user', drug use was discussed by service-users as an interruption of the flows of desire. The accounts above show that the recovery assemblage does not come to cover up the cracks but to acknowledge them, to explore how boundaries lead to the re-emergence of the interrupted flows of desire in a safe space, where they can be negotiated without threatening the connections that hold the recovery assemblage together. The desire of becoming-other through substances has been explored as an individual desire that, when unable to connect with other bodies, leads to undesired destratifications. In the recovery assemblage, the desire of becoming-other through substances is not challenged through medicalised perceptions on what constitutes 'healthy choices', but through the production of alternate orderings where connections with other human and non-human bodies become possible and open up lines of flight. The concept of boundaries in the recovery assemblage contributes towards this direction by operating as symbolic constraints, not imposed from the outside, but organically produced from within, as elements that do not come to block but to enhance a body's capacity to make connections and act.

Within this framework, setting boundaries is a personal matter, for example:

> At 18 [ano] I understood that I have to set the boundaries, my personal boundaries, with others but also with myself.

And it is also a practical and symbolic commitment to the collective:

> At the beginning I was breaching them [the boundaries]. In general I had a complete lack of boundaries. When they were talking about boundaries I couldn't understand what they were talking about. I couldn't understand it in practice. When they said that's a boundary, I could understand. [I could understand that] Abstaining from substances is a boundary. Keeping the boundaries, especially in the pious way that it happens in the residential stage ... for me, it was gradually, after a period of 2–3 months that I saw their deeper meaning, that boundaries are completely symbolic. Some things are also practical because otherwise a group of people can't function. If we don't clean we can't live in a humane and healthy environment. But especially the symbolic boundaries, they made me think in ways that I hadn't thought before ... For me, and I had done it, hiding it [breaching a boundary], the guilt, it's very much like the feeling of hiding a relapse. But sharing, and opening up about breaching a boundary relieves, not as a confession, but in the sense of the commitment that I won't breach it again, and the trust, that you open up, you talk about it with the therapists and they don't punish you, they just ask you to not do it again and there's a relationship of trust and for me that's unprecedented. I never had relationships of trust before.

Boundaries in the account above do not operate as preventative measures that could lead to punishment, but as symbolic and practical links that enable the production of affective flows and hold the recovery assemblage together. These small gestures of commitment to one's self and others reflect de la Bellacasa's (2010) practices of everyday ethos transformation, 'ethical doings' that do not define a code of conduct or a normative definition of right and wrong, without though implying,

> *that the ethos is unruly. An ethos is marked by constraints ... This is different than explaining ethos by behaving according to pre-existent norms and conventions that sort out the good and the bad, the true and the false; or of explaining 'choice' as the action of the objective self-reliant individuals in a given situation.*
>
> (de la Bellacasa, 2010: 152)

What boundaries help keep together 'is not a city of honest men and women but a heterogeneous collective' (Stengers, 2010: 52), where the desire of becoming-other is reinvested. The service-users' narratives account for the understanding of boundaries as affective expressions of care, becoming collectively. Family structures are also discussed as formations where care is expressed through the identification of boundaries:

> *Since I was a child I didn't know what a boundary means. I would study until late and nobody bothered, I was leaving the house for many hours, there was no schedule, no boundary, I'm talking about simple things but actually very important.*

The recovery assemblage comes to address this need through the provision of a daily structure, and most importantly through the encouragement of the practical and symbolic commitment of all service-users and staff to the relationships built within the recovery assemblage. As discussed through the exploration of the material assemblage of recovery, the clash between using time and recovery time was collectively addressed by the workers and the service-users. The daily structure and the boundaries that accompany the residential stage of 18 ano are an extension of the caring practices deployed by Genie. While in the drug assemblage, destratifications blocked the connections between bodies, in the recovery assemblage, conflict is one of the components that hold the assemblage together, enhancing the affective resources that emerge. This juxtaposition between the connections produced 'inside' and 'outside' the recovery assemblage takes us back to what was earlier discussed as a 'corrective' experience.

> *We want to believe that as a therapeutic team we constitute a corrective experience in the family relations of each service-user ... Our aim isn't to*

replace the family, but to show how in a group, like the family is, or like the programme here, it is possible that things function differently. With rights, responsibilities, equality, freedom of speech, respect, care, and if there's also love, even better.

It is important to look closely at how this 'corrective' experience is talked about. Unlike discourses that position the 'correction' of the individual in the focus of attention, in the recovery assemblage it is not the service-user that has to be 'corrected', but the experiences that they have had of social structures, like family formations and other institutions, leading to the destratification of their desires. In doing so, the recovery assemblage does not replace existing social structures; it creates a sociality where *things can function differently*. Doing things otherwise does not become possible through the 'right' choices made by individuals, but through practices of care and affective flows that hold this heterogeneous collective together. That is where the importance of talking about the recovery space as an assemblage lies. Shifting the focus of attention away from the service-users' individual choices, the manuals on the application of recovery models and the responsibilisation of drug workers, the assemblage addresses the recovery experience as a matter of the collective and not the individual, concerned with the ways in which human and non-human components come together to form safe and caring environments.

Therefore, an ethics of care comes into being in the recovery assemblage. Duff, drawing on Mol (2008), argues that an ethics of care emphasises

> *the everyday practices, procedures, relationships and rhetorical strategies by which ethical problems are identified, debated, managed and sometimes resolved ... ethical problems ought to be regarded as the product of specific failures to develop and sustain relationships of trust, compassion, fairness and respect among the parties to such problems.*
>
> (Duff, 2015: 86)

The ethics of care of the recovery assemblage focus on the identification of the ethical problems – the forces that interrupted the development and sustainability of relationships of trust, compassion, fairness and respect – that blocked the desire of becoming-other, and produce corrective experiences through the everyday practices, relationships and boundaries that render recovery a shared matter of care. I will now discuss how these ethics of care generate the affective resource of hope, unblocking the desire of becoming-other.

Becoming hopeful

I just took photos of the ones that I thought were relevant to recovery. And that's obvious, don't give up there's hope thing, obviously someone else did

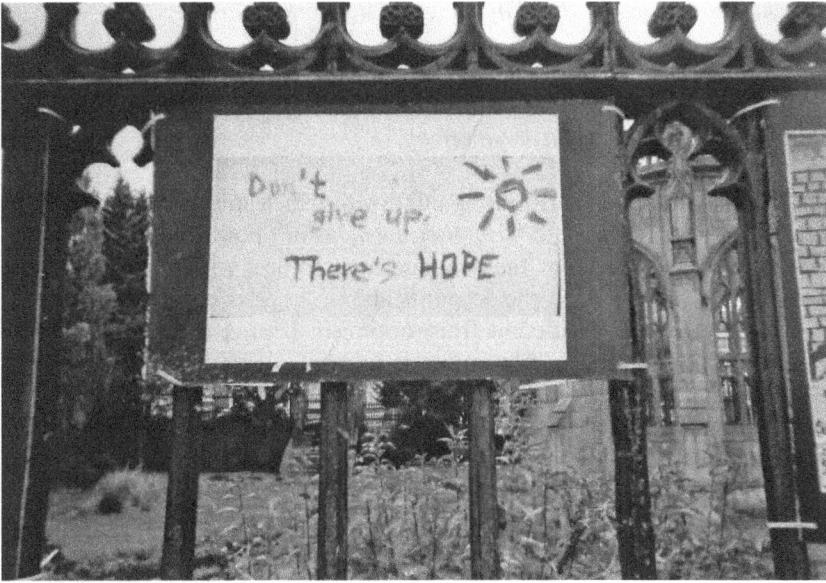

Figure 6.1 Don't give up, there's hope, Liverpool.

that but that's kind of a sort of a keep going attitude thing I was trying to get there.

For the photographer of the picture above, the message *'don't give up there's hope'* is *obviously* relevant to recovery. This certainty potentially derives from his own experience of recovery, combined with theoretical and empirical associations between recovery and hope (Glassman et al., 2013; Maddock and Hallam, 2010; Mathis et al., 2009). The question that I am initially concerned with in relation to recovery and hope, is not whether recovery generates hope, but *where in time* does hope happen? Is hope an affective expression of one's *present* (Alacovska, 2018) state of being, or is it an investment for the *future* (Kuehn and Corrigan, 2013; Mische, 2009)? I then argue that the generation of hope as an affective resource becoming in the recovery assemblage is timeless, in the sense that while it derives from present practices, it expands life possibilities beyond the temporality and territoriality of the recovery assemblage.

Following the accounts of some of the service-users, it could be argued that hope matters as an affective resource that renders the present enjoyable:

the past's gone, I don't know what the future has in store, just keep it in the moment, deal with it, enjoy what you're doing now if it's good, even if it's shit, pardon my language but you know you face it, deal with it the best way you can, and that's what I'm doing and it's working for me.

So I'm putting a lot in, I make sure I do that, but I do it because I want to and I'm enjoying what I'm doing and also I'm getting a hell of a lot out of it as well, so I feel good about myself.

The past is gone and the future is unknown, which means that we are left with the present; we have to '*keep it in the moment*'. Following this thinking, hope is our ability to enjoy the here and now, to deal with whatever comes, in the best way we can. In the accounts above, 'hope is *not* connected to an expected success; it is different from optimism because it is placed in the *present*' (Massumi, 2002: 211, emphasis in original). Hope in that sense is generated and experienced through the connections that become possible in the recovery assemblage. For other service-users hope is associated with the expansion of future life possibilities:

The people, the workers, you know what I mean? They show you, how can I put it, they show you, I can't think of the word, they show you I'd say love, they show you a bit of love, a bit of kindness, a bit of help, a bit of future, looking into the future.

What the recovery assemblage offers is a taste of the affective resources (*a bit of love, a bit of kindness, a bit of help, a bit of future*) that render a future beyond the recovery assemblage possible. Hope emerges when one has enough resources in her quiver in order to connect with other assemblages. Thinking of hope as an affective resource to be materialised in the future, means that it 'anticipates that something indeterminate has *not-yet-become* … an intuitive understanding that hope matters because it discloses the creation of potentiality or possibility' (Anderson, 2006: 733, emphasis in original). The danger of understanding hope as a good way of being that has 'still not become', renders the 'present haunted by the fact that the something good that exceeds it has yet to take place' (ibid: 743).

However, in our thinking with becoming, the relationship between the present and the future is complicated. Accordingly, thinking hope with becoming explores how the affective practices becoming in the assemblage, expand the possibilities for connections with other assemblages in a future yet to come. Becoming is not just in the present, nor an investment for the future; becoming is all there is (Biehl and Locke, 2010), the enactment of a body that is never fixed or stable but endlessly shifting with the assemblages it affects and is affected by. Therefore, the hope generated in the recovery assemblage is neither fixed in the present, nor the future. Becoming hopeful reflects the affective resources generated in the recovery assemblage through the connections produced, *and* the possibility of a future that extends these connections to other assemblages. According to Stengers:

> *hope is the difference between probability and possibility. If we follow probability there is no hope, just a calculated anticipation authorised by the world as it is. But to 'think' is to create possibility against probability. It doesn't mean hope for one or another thing or as a calculated attitude, but to try and feel and put into words a possibility for becoming.*
>
> (Stengers, 2002: 245, emphasis in original)

Through the connections produced in the recovery assemblage, the possibility of becoming is created. The question shifts from when and how hope happens, to 'what can a body do when it becomes hopeful? What capacities, and capabilities, are enabled?' (Anderson, 2006: 734). Through the following field notes I unfold hope and its becoming as an affective expression of the connections that traverse the theatre group of 18 ano, expanding the field of possibilities in the present and future:

A couple of months after completing my fieldwork, I went back to visit the theatre group of 18 ano. At the time the group was intensively rehearsing for Mike Kane's 'Boy with the suitcase' as there was only one week left until the premier of the play. A couple of hours before the rehearsal the main facilitator of the group and director of the play called to warn me that the rehearsal would be intense as a service-user who was playing one of the main characters had broken one of the fundamental boundaries of the programme and consequently she wouldn't be part of the play anymore. Another service-user would have to replace her and learn all the words within a week. All members of the group were distressed, nervous and disappointed. When I arrived, as it always happens at the beginning of each session, we sat in a circle to discuss changes and updates. The main facilitator and drama therapist appeared to be in a good and cheerful mood, he avoided discussing the details of what had happened with the service-user that had to leave the group and quickly asked who wanted to replace her. A volunteer was found, and we started rehearsing some parts of the play. Throughout the rehearsal, the facilitator was running up and down directing them, and within half an hour from starting, the whole group was in a good mood and the replacement of the role in question *did not only seem probable but possible*. At the end of each group a 'check-out' takes place, where all members share their feelings. At that point, the facilitator expressed his sadness about the service-user that had left the group but also stressed out how important it is to find a way to keep going. When going around the circle one of the service-users thanked him for everything he had done for them that day; for cheering them up through his sense of humour, for making the replacement of the role possible and for motivating them; for generating hope.

I left thinking that what the group had accomplished that day was to become hopeful *with* anger and disappointment; it resisted becoming blocked. The becoming hopeful body of the group rendered possible the simultaneous negotiation of a series of negative feelings – the sadness and potentially the anger for the exclusion of one of the members, and the anxiety and uncertainty about the outcome of the play. Although the emphasis is on the drama therapist's ability to navigate all these feelings, hope was becoming, as the rehearsal evolved, through the connections created between the members, and with their facilitators, as well as with the play itself. Hope in other words was affectively generated through the connections of the human and non-human components that constituted the assemblage of the specific theatre group. Enacting hope in that occasion was not only a way to make the play possible, but to expand the possibilities of life overall.

Most importantly, the group managed to *enjoy* the rehearsal. The importance of joy in the engagement with the recovery assemblage was also emphasised by one of the service-users above: *I'm enjoying what I'm doing.* Massumi, drawing on Spinoza, discusses joy as affirmation, 'an assuming of the body of its potentials, its assuming of a posture that intensifies its powers of existence. The moment of joy is the co-presence of those potentials, in the context of a bodily becoming' (Massumi, 2002: 241). Joy is the affective resource that renders the experience of hope possible in the present, as well as important for the future. Joy, through the intensification of a body's powers of existence, extends its power of acting, expands the possibilities of life, renders becoming hopeful possible. In the theatre group hope was generated when the group members became able to laugh, to enjoy the rehearsal, to enjoy the present. The fact that the present could be enjoyed, with all its difficulties, generated hope for the group's upcoming performance. Generated in the present, and enhancing a body's capacity to act in the present and future, hope does not have a particular content or end point; 'it's a desire for more life, or for more to life' (Massumi, 2002: 242).

This enactment of hope and its extension to other assemblages traverses all caring practices of the recovery assemblage. The provision of care is entangled with the service-users' future becomings, as these are made possible through the connections and the negotiation of problems and obstacles within the recovery space:

> *What I saw at 18 [ano] from the beginning is that things are humane, that they can be talked about and that maybe a solution will be found.*

According to the therapeutic principles of 18 ano, the usefulness of psychotherapy lies in the fact that it is 'discursive'. As discussed in relation to the establishment of boundaries, '*things can be talked about*', and by talking '*a solution might be found*'. The process of finding solutions refers to the problems encountered within as well as beyond the recovery assemblage.

Becoming hopeful in the account above is enacted through the belief that if one talks, they will be heard, and in turn being heard practically means that a system of care is mobilised to collectively look for a solution.

Throughout this chapter, the emphasis has been on the transitions that the connections produced in the recovery assemblage render possible. 'Turning up' for an assessment appointment necessitated a transition from using time to recovery time, a transition that becomes desirable as the connection between the service-users and the workers evolve through the provision of care that extends beyond the territoriality of the recovery space (see for example the practice of checking-in). Accordingly, hope emerges from the '*transitions that take place during spatially and temporally distributed encounters*' (Anderson, 2006: 735, emphasis in original). In the theatre group, in the psychotherapeutic encounter, over the phone, new relations are established, disclosing 'a point of contingency within a present space – time' (ibid: 744). It is through these connections that a possibility of becoming is created (Stengers, 2002: 245), the possibility of hope as an affective resource 'that provides a dynamic imperative *to action* in that it enables bodies to *go on*' (Anderson, 2006: 744, emphasis in original) and expand their life possibilities beyond the recovery assemblage.

The social assemblage

I now focus on the social assemblage, starting from the sociality produced within the recovery space and then moving on to investigate how the desires and affects generated extend to other social assemblages.

The photograph below, taken by a service-user and accompanied by the discussion it initiated, depicts one of the guest houses of 18 ano, a house where service-users live collectively after they have completed the residential stage of the programme. The aim of this type of accommodation is to assist them in their transition from the recovery assemblage to other social assemblages, and it mainly covers housing needs of service-users that are either not from Athens, or do not have another, safe place of residence. All spaces (living room, kitchen, bathroom and rooms) are shared and it is the responsibility of the residents to run all the housekeeping activities, as well as maintain the therapeutic boundaries of the programme.

The discussion that follows took place during our group analysis of the visual material produced:

Photographer: That's actually very personal. I mean, I'm showing you the toilet that I'm using ... and lots of people find it difficult to photograph their personal spaces.

Participant 1: ... I think that's the most successful part (of the photograph), that it can combine the old, the timeless of the camera and you don't know the time, it can be now, it can be the past, it can be a lot of years ago.

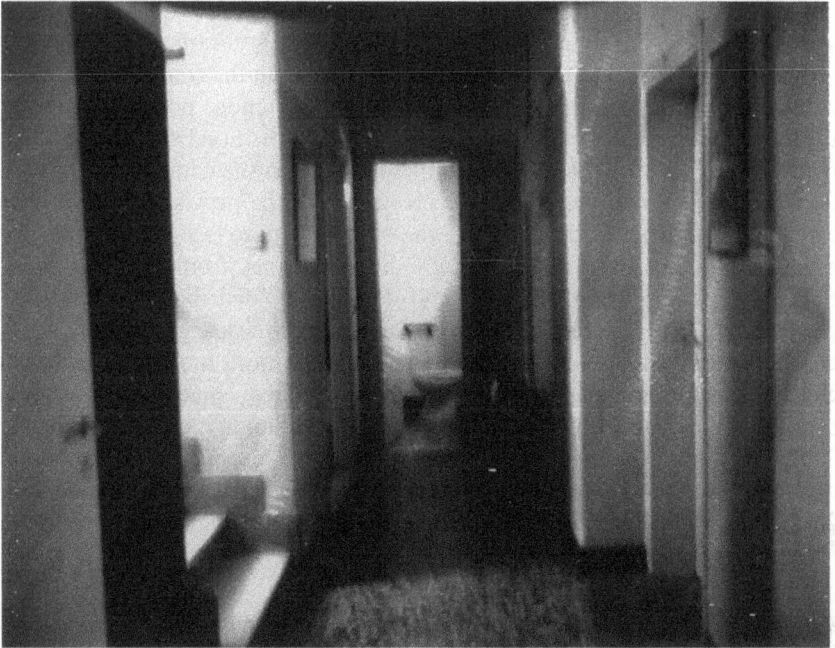

Figure 6.2 A personal space, Athens.

*Photographer: Also, in this photo let's say, for me that took it, it's a very
personal space but who else might have been there before, who might have
passed by? It's not just me, so many people have passed and I'm just one
of them.*

*Participant 2: I want to say that I like it because it creates questions and it can
take each person at a different place. It lets the imagination go wild.*

This analysis of the photograph begins with the photographer describing it as
a '*very personal space*'. The conversation then focuses on the different times
and spaces that are visually presented. The photographer has used a vintage
Polaroid camera, producing '*timeless*' black and white pictures. The description of the photograph as '*timeless*' refers to the type of the camera used, as
well as to the space captured, a personal space for the photographer but also
a shared one, not only with the people that lived at the guest house at the time
but with everyone else that '*might have passed by*'. The discussion ends with
another participant observing that the photograph '*can take each person at a
different place*'.

This way of thinking with time and space reflects Foucault's description of heterotopias as 'capable of juxtaposing in a single real place several spaces, several sites that are in themselves incompatible' (Foucault, 1986: 27). The guest house is a real space where personal sites are juxtaposed with shared ones. While this recovery space is personal in its everyday use and the ways in which it is experienced, it also connects all the bodies that have inhabited it, as for all of them it has been a temporal, 'a transitional moment or point of passage' (Hetherington, 1997: 18) from the recovery to other social assemblages. The individual histories are shared through conviviality, rendering it a social space linked 'to slices of time' (Foucault, 1986: 27), slices of personal time, shared time and timelessness. This 'sharing' of the recovery space is linked to the investment of desire. While the individual desire of becoming-other through substances, led to the body becoming blocked, the desire within the recovery assemblage begins 'from a multiplicity of investments which traverse persons' (Colebrook, 2001: 141). The affective relations discussed earlier in this chapter are also an intrinsic component of this social experience of the recovery space as

> *[i]n affect, we are never alone. That's because affects in Spinoza's defin-*
> *ition are basically ways of* connecting, *to others and to other situations …*
> *With intensified affect comes a stronger sense of embeddedness in a larger*
> *field of life – a heightened sense of belonging, with other people and to other*
> *places.*
>
> (Massumi, 2002: 214, emphasis in original)

The recovery space has been discussed as one of 'otherness', a space where affective practices of care reassemble the destratified flows of desire and render a becoming-other possible. The recovery assemblage *makes a difference* by producing alternate orderings that 'do not sit in isolation as reservoirs of freedom, emancipation or resistance; they coexist, combine and connect' (Johnson, 2013: 800) within the societies where they come into being. The link between Foucault's heterotopias and the Deleuzo–Guattarian assemblage lies in the lines of flight that the heterotopia of recovery opens up, 'what Deleuze calls a line of subjectivity and fracture' (Johnson, 2006: 86). Within the recovery assemblage, where safety is enacted through the provision of care, subjectivities are fractured and reassembled. Destratifications are not sidelined but constitutive of a becoming-well process that revisits the desire of becoming-other (McLeod, 2017). In what follows I discuss the recovery and art group activities that take place within the recovery assemblage, and how, through their exploration, power relations can be thought about differently in spaces that 'light up an imaginary field, a set of relations that are not separate from dominant structures and ideology, but go against the grain and offer lines of flight' (Johnson, 2006: 87).

The recovery group

The structured recovery group holds a special and central space in the recovery assemblage. Although the affective forces that define the recovery assemblage are present in all its different layers and moments, it is in the group setting that they are being articulated, enacted, negotiated and reflected upon. According to group facilitators in both Liverpool and Athens, uniqueness and unexpectedness are two elements that define all types of recovery groups. They are unique as each group session is a process of becoming, creating affective flows between the members of the group that can never be replicated in exactly the same way, and unexpected because the contribution of each group member can never be predicted in advance. As explained by one of the art therapists of 18 ano:

> *The main part of how the group is set depends on the guys [service-users], so each group is different. Each group has its own dynamics, there's no pro-cut in the treatment of addiction.*

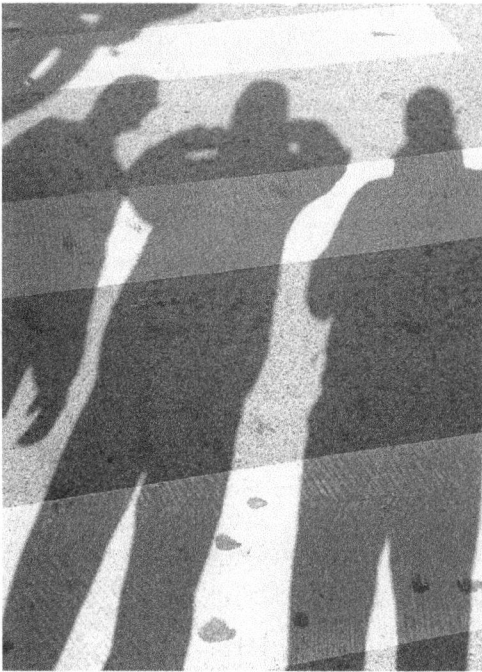

Figure 6.3 The group, Athens.

> *Here, I was trying to capture the group, that I'm not alone in all this. We're not alone*

The aim of the group in the recovery assemblage is to allow for encounters between bodies in such a way that the relations that emerge form a body with increased affective capacity (McLeod, 2017: 17). Guattari's work with groups provides a valuable insight to the potentialities of the group in the recovery assemblage. The group setting has been studied by Guattari as a *collective assemblage of enunciation* (Guattari and Rolnik, 2008). While it appears to be a closed and limited structure, 'Guattari does not stop at the "group-as-a-whole" as the outer limit of the group therapeutic practice. There is always "a beyond" that takes therapy into the wider social field: wider than the person, wider than the family and wider than the collective' (Slater, 2013).

The first step towards the becoming of this collective assemblage of enunciation is the gradual transition from becoming isolated to 'becoming part of':

> *The fact that you walk into a room and you see that it's not just you who has been going through all that is very important … It makes you softer.*

'*Walking into a room*' and '*becoming softer*' reflects the physical effort required and the affective transformation that follows during a body's initial engagement with a recovery group. Through this transformation, the enunciation of suffering becomes possible, not as an individual experience anymore, but as one collectively articulated:

> *Because when you're drinking on your own, you think you're the only person who's feeling like this and you're the only person who's going through this kind of torment, and the only person who is suffering the way I was suffering. And then you come to Genie or somewhere like Genie, and you find out there's lots and lots of people are suffering, some with drink, some with drugs and some with anything else maybe, other problems, but there's lots of people going through similar things. I'm not alone and I'm not you know forced to remain on my own and just you know get on with it.*

The decision made possible within the group, to not '*just get on with it*', but to stay with it, opens up a field of encounters that render the group not just a sum of individual subjectivities (Guattari and Rolnik, 2008: 51), but a body with increased capacity to act:

> *Being involved with the groups, the recovery groups, it's great just to listen to other people as well and being able to connect in that way and relate it with, you know there's a lot of stuff that gets mentioned from certain people, well everyone really who takes part, and there's always someone, if not all of them, where you can think, yeah, I know exactly where you're coming from there. And you know when I'm given my opportunity to you know say my bit, put it across there, I'll get that back as well and it makes you feel part of something special then, you know, it's like a community.*

The account above reflects on the connections made possible within the recovery group and how contributing to these connections through sharing personal experiences '*makes you feel part of something special*'. Following on from previous chapters, where it was not the substance as such that formed the core of the participants' narratives, but their desire of becoming-other, accordingly, the recovery group goes beyond an exchange of experiences of drug use and recovery. While becoming with the group, the desire of 'becoming part of' flows, leading to the production of a social assemblage that commences from the recovery group but extends beyond it:

> *Throughout my life I always said I'll make it on my own, until I realised that I can't do anything on my own ... every time I was hearing the word 'group' I was like as if my own pain isn't enough, I'm gonna have the other's too. But eventually, when I shut up and started listening to the others [members of the group] with some I identified with, with others I could feel their pain and then I got 'unlocked' and started talking, said things that I'd never told anyone and through this a relationship of trust was built.*

While the recovery group provides a space for suffering and pain to be shared, it also enhances a body's capacity to act in connection with others, to not '*just get on with it*' but to become 'unlocked' and build relationships of trust. One becomes 'unlocked' not by offloading their pain, but by becoming with each other's pain, rendering suffering not an individual problem, but a shared one. This process of becoming with each other extends beyond the group's collective assemblage of enunciation, enhancing the possibilities of other social assemblages that the members of the group inhabit.

The flows produced when the members of the group go beyond their individual subjectivities and operate as a body with increased affective capacity is what Guattari refers to as 'transversality'.

> *Transversality in the group is a dimension opposite and complementary to the structures that generate pyramidal hierarchization and sterile ways of transmitting messages. Transversality is the unconscious source of action in the group, going beyond the objective laws on which it is based, carrying the group's desire.*

(Guattari, 1984: 22)

The recovery group becomes a machine 'capable of sweeping away earlier stratifications and creating the conditions necessary for desire to function in a new way' (Guattari, 1984: 218). As will be discussed further on, the deterritorialisations that become in the recovery group extend beyond it and carry the group's desire of becoming-other beyond the recovery assemblage, into assemblages of work, family and other social formations and institutions.

Art groups

Drawing on the accounts and experiences of service-users and workers, it has been demonstrated that the recovery space does not operate as a storage of therapeutic tools, available to be 'applied' to service-users. Conversely, it is produced as an assemblage where the treatment practices flow, enabling connections and new becomings. As explained by one of the therapists of 18 ano:

> *Therapy is a team work, it's the resultant of many things, painting, drama-therapy, psychotherapy, nursing, medicine, it's all together, it's a pie, it's a puzzle.*

Accordingly, art therapy is not practised as an alternative or additional recovery method, but instead constitutes an intrinsic component of the recovery assemblage. Although the theory behind the deployment of artistic practice differs in 18 ano and Genie, for both services the creative groups complement the recovery ones by opening up new flows of desire:

> *Art helps people to find solutions using their creativity ... Creativity is how you're going to make this table more beautiful so that you can sit and feel good in your own space. By learning to paint you learn a whole world, a language, you learn to see, then you have other expectations ... it [art] opens up the possibility to see differently, to live differently, to invest emotionally in a different way. This is what art can bring in a therapeutic space.*

This art therapist of 18 ano does not describe art as an additional skill but as a vehicle that opens up ways of experiencing – seeing, living, feeling – '*differently*'. The experience of producing art in the recovery space, enables a *different investment of desire*. According to one of Genie's workers, in some cases it opens up a path, when all other routes appear to be blocked:

> *Sometimes you can't express exactly how you're really feeling through talking and again because they [service-users] maybe talked so much throughout their lives and feel like nobody listened.*

It is very common to frame art in recovery as a different means of expression; as a way to say creatively what one cannot say with words. What is interesting about the quote above, is the acknowledgment that there will be service-users that do not *want* to talk, because they feel that when they did '*nobody listened*'. This view adds an extra weight to art therapy, as a way to include in recovery those who would otherwise be excluded, those that do not experience talking therapy as a way to unblock their flows of desire. Overall, artistic practice in recovery contributes to the becoming of a social assemblage that does not operate as a closed system with specific norms, but remains flexible and open, constantly in search of the practices that will render it as inclusive as possible.

When discussing the generation of hope in the affective recovery assemblage, it was demonstrated, through the description of one of the rehearsals of the theatre group of 18 ano, how joy enhances hope. The following account of a member of staff of Genie takes us back to the same argument:

> I think one of the big positives for art therapy is people are doing what they want to do. So it's something they enjoy doing and if we can enhance the recovery journey through something they enjoy doing, I think it's a huge positive.

The social assemblage of recovery does not only address a collective enunciation of suffering, but also a shared experience of hope, joy and safety. The art group, an intrinsic component of the sociality of the recovery assemblage, attends equally to the sufferings that remain untold, as well as to the dreams, hopes and aspirations of the future becomings of its members. Zontou (2013), researcher and practitioner of drama therapy who has worked with the theatre group of 18 ano, addresses, from another epistemological perspective, this multiplicity of affects, as it unfolds through the symbolic potential of the plays chosen to be performed by the group. Drawing on her engagement with social and applied theatre (Boal, 1995; Cohen-Cruz, 2012; Nicholson, 2014), Zontou's analysis follows the new life possibilities that emerge as the service-users become with the roles they have chosen to embody:

> the directors choose plays that have the potential to not only symbolise and reflect upon the participants' personal experiences and fears, but also their dreams and expectations. The idea of symbolisation and the use of metaphors have a central role in 18 ANO's approach, since it is believed that, by activating the process of symbolisation the individuals will learn to confer new meanings onto objects and concepts, and that eventually this might allow them to conceptualise and construct their lives on a new basis ... participation in theatre allows the participants to move beyond what they have already experienced, by introducing them to something different and new.
>
> (Zontou, 2013: 264–265)

In Zontou's analysis symbolisation does not only refer to the connections made between the dramatic roles performed and the lived experiences of the service-users/actors, but also to the new becomings rendered possible through the whole process. As a component of the transitional and transformative recovery assemblage, the theatre group of 18 ano symbolically transforms 'the participants from being an addict, strange, deviant to being a 'protagonist' on the theatrical stage' (Zontou, 2013: 266). Following this line of thought, and returning to the earlier point made about the role of artistic practice in the social recovery assemblage, art is not just there to increase the 'recovery time'; to keep people in recovery busy and away from substances, but to create its own 'chains of decoding and deterritorialization that serve as the foundation for desiring-machines, and make them function' (Deleuze and Guattari, 1977: 368).

I now investigate how creativity builds a bridge between the therapeutic environment and the social, enabling connections between the recovery assemblage and other assemblages beyond the recovery space.

Recovery in the community

While engaging with recovery services, service-users collectively renegotiate their positionality within the social field. This renegotiation, enabled by the mediation of the recovery assemblage as a transitional, safe and hopeful space, focuses on how desire in the social field can be differently invested. In previous chapters it was discussed how one becomes a drug user when the assemblages within which they operate block the flows of desire of becoming-other. Within the recovery assemblage, the desire of becoming-other is unblocked through affective relationships that generate safety, hope and a shared subjectivity. 'Returning' to the social field, service-users are called to confront the (lack of) connections that blocked their individual desires in the first place, and to fight for the continuation of the flow of the desires produced in the recovery assemblage. The shared subjectivity though emerging in the recovery assemblage 'is not situated in the individual field, but in the process of social and material production' (Guattari and Rolnik, 2008: 45); it does not return to an empty field awaiting to become through new investments of desires, but to a social field immediately invested by the historically determined product of desire (Deleuze and Guattari, 1977: 29).

In order to follow the trajectories of the service-users as they move on to other assemblages, and to address the specificities of the investment of desire in the socialities within which they are called to operate, I examine separately how the recovery assemblage extends to other assemblages in Athens and in Liverpool. By exploring the production of sociality through the lived experiences of people in recovery, I address Duff's call for analyses that do not 'naturalise' sociality 'as innately healthy or therapeutic, leaving unresolved the question of how social interaction is mediated in a social field, and how sociality actually supports recovery' (2014a: 100). Discussing social reintegration and the cultivation of social ties as unconditionally 'positive' does little to challenge policymaking tendencies like 'new recovery', a paradigm of treatment promoting freedom, choice, transformation and new aspirations that has become a prominent feature of drug policy in the UK, Australia and elsewhere during the past decade (Fomiatti, Moore and Fraser, 2019: 527). The 'new recovery's' 'enactment of the social underpins and reinforces a hierarchical logic in which individual subjects are obliged to recover by controlling and changing their social environments through enterprise and activity' (ibid: 528). This perception of the social does not take into consideration the mechanisms that blocked the service-users' flow of desire in the first place, and describes it instead as a field of opportunities that the 'recovered', responsible individuals have to make the best of. This practice is in conflict with the social becoming enabled through connection that enhance the collective body's capacity to act.

Following the service-users' narratives, I explore how their encounters with other assemblages transform their affective orientations, either by enhancing their power of acting or diminishing it. Deleuze, through his reading of Spinoza, argues that encounters are 'good' for the affected body when they enter into composition with it and 'bad' when they decompose it, accordingly increasing or diminishing its power of acting or force of existing (Deleuze, 1988: 50). While encounters between service-users and other socialities are experienced as 'good' when mediated by the recovery assemblage, in its absence such encounters can produce insecurities and fears associated with social expectations and the lack of supportive mechanisms that prevent isolation.

Athens

In 2017, when I was conducting fieldwork in Athens, Greece had been for almost ten years in what was called a 'financial' and eventually also 'social' crisis. Although 18 ano managed to survive the 'crisis' without having to close any of its services, austerity politics led to extensive cuts of the budget of the national health system (where 18 ano administratively belongs); the wages of the workers significantly reduced, and the conditions under which therapy was delivered deteriorated.

As commented by one of the therapists of 18 ano, this degradation of the public health system led to a series of practical issues that affected the daily operation of the service:

> the quality of the food [provided for the service-users during the residential stage] has deteriorated ... Nothing gets fixed and the workers have to improvise, from the windows that don't close properly to the lack of pens and files for example ... When Loverdos[2] was Health Minister, I remember meeting mothers with their kids in a freezing room.

The impoverishment of recovery and other health services was not only attributed to a lack of funds, but as a psychologist of 18 ano put it 'there is always violence from the state to the people, which escalates during times of crises'. The response of 18 ano to this state violence came through the mobilisation of its political and activist reflexes that have accompanied its history. During those years, service-users together with members of staff joined the growing (at the time), anti-austerity social movement, through for example their participation in anti-fascist events, the organisation of discussions on addiction in collaboration with squats and social centres, and their active support of the occupation of the headquarters of the national broadcaster (ERT)[3] when the government at the time attempted to shut it down overnight. The activist past of 18 ano and its participation in the political assemblages becoming as a response to the crisis were also reflected in the continuous provision of care, besides the practical difficulties and degradation of the healthcare services. The following statement from one of the therapists of 18 ano is indicative of the ways that collective political practices were embodied by the recovery assemblage:

There was a lot of insecurity, that's for sure. But there was also at the same time a dynamic tendency, in relation to what in the end can one achieve through collective practices. We were all (members of staff) united, not just in relation to the political framework and how to protect the organisation or claim the resources needed, but also in the social dialogue taking place. Once for example I had an appointment with a mother (service-user) that told me 'I have 5 euros and my kid is 5 years old. How am I gonna feed it?' There, on the one hand we had to talk about the foods with the highest nutritional value, the potential of improvisation and the need of the collaboration between the mothers in order to set up solidarity networks. It was this social net that was being weaved during those times in order to provide a multilevelled support to the organisation, the service-users, the workers, that had to establish their positions in a health system that needs to exist not just for some people to have a job, but because it provides a necessary service.

18 ano, constituted of approximately 33 services, including 2 residential recovery services for women (of which one is for mothers and their children) and 3 for men, and 5 guest houses where all living costs are covered, is admittedly a significant expense for the national health system. The workers of the organisation take pride in having managed to keep all these services open, as explained by one of the 18 ano therapists:

It's unprecedented in the crisis-stricken Greece and incredible poverty for one to meet, as part of the national health [system], a service that [one] would imagine [would only exist] in a Scandinavian state. The quality of the provided services is that good!

The connection of 18 ano with the socialities extending beyond the recovery space is to a great extent ensured through the participation of its art groups in various events. The pottery group, jewellery-making group and art group frequently exhibit the artefacts produced at various neighbourhoods' events and annual festivals like the anti-racist festival that takes place once per year in Athens. A special place in this engagement with the social is held by the theatre group, whose primary aim through their performances is to engage wider audiences in discussions on addiction, helping to destigmatise drug use and to promote social inclusion for people in recovery. Across the years they have performed in neighbourhood squares, community centres, children's hospitals, residential care homes for the elderly, art festivals and prisons.

The plays performed, chosen by the facilitators of the group, focus on challenging 'the social stereotypes and misconception frequently associated with addiction' (Zontou, 2013: 262). According to Zontou's, experience of working empirically with 18 ano, the participants of the group do not reproduce narratives of redemption and salvation, but through the dramatic characters that they perform they open up a space 'in between' their personal realities and fiction, and it is in these moments of in-betweeness that the audience is invited to imagine the possibility of a hopeful and positive future in their lives (Zontou, 2013: 271). Additionally, the group follows a 'role claim model':

According to this model, each participant is required to select the dramatic role that they would like to perform and explain why they should get it. They are asked to choose a role which would allow them to express and reflect upon their personal issues and background. This process has a double function: firstly, it ensures that equal opportunities are given to each participant – gaining in this way the ownership of the process and become responsible for that aspect of the performances; and secondly, the participants are given the opportunity to ask for the dramatic role of their choice, allowing them in this way to develop an aesthetic distance between their lives and their characters' lives.

(Zontou, 2013: 266)

The affective flows produced within the theatre group and their extension to other socialities, provide an indicative example of the connections that become possible within the recovery assemblage, enhancing a body's capacity to act, and leading to the production of flows of desire that extend to other assemblages. More specifically, the facilitators' choice of the play to be performed, is the outcome of their encounter with the service-users until that point. The affective assemblage produced renders the facilitators capable of identifying a play that can enhance the connections made within the recovery assemblage, and renders the service-users trustful of the facilitators' capacity to do so. Further, the 'role claim' approach is the first point of contact between the recovery assemblage and other assemblages. Through this process, the service-users produce a link between the affective flows that have been shared in the recovery space and the affective flows that form the assemblage of the chosen play. In that sense, the recovery body connects to another, fictional body which, although existing outside the recovery assemblage, experiences situations and feelings the service-user identifies with in a symbolic fashion. A series of connections is subsequently produced: the recovering body connects with the fictional body, fictional and real characters mingle during the process of the rehearsal, and the service-users explore novel affective flows within a group that keeps shifting between reality and fiction. Overall, these connections enhance the group's capacity to act, through a collective enactment of the desire of becoming-other and extending this desire outside the recovery assemblage. On the stage, the recovering body becomes other not through the loss of one-self, but through complex and multilayered connections. It is through these connections that the desire of becoming-other is unblocked, and through its communication to the audience that the recovery assemblage extends to another sociality. The performance produces a social assemblage, becoming with the recovering bodies *and* the audience, increasing the capacity of all the bodies involved to affect and be affected.

I want to now return to the group's rejection of the reproduction of narratives of redemption and salvation, by going back to my own experience of working with the theatre group of 18 ano. During the rehearsals, it is very often discussed that the aim is not to get the audience's recognition simply because the actors are in recovery, but due to the quality of their performance, their ability to connect with the characters they are performing and to symbolically communicate their own realities through fiction. Therefore, rehearsals are demanding and intense, usually three hours long once or twice per week. Earlier in this chapter, when discussing the generation of hope as an affective practice, field notes from the theatre group were shared to demonstrate how joy and humour can shift what appears to be a hopeless situation into a hopeful one. This aspect of recovery is not only communicated within the group, but also in the engagement of service-users with socialities extending beyond the recovery assemblage. Very often, after a public performance, a discussion follows between the actors and the audience. These discussions can occasionally get emotional, when members of the group share their experience of the recovery process and their connection with the characters they have chosen to embody. Following a performance of 'Medea', I was attending one such discussion that got some of the audience and actors in tears. When closing the event, one of the members of the group said that although he identified with the emotions shared, he wanted to stress out that rehearsals can also be fun, and usually after they finish, all service-users go together for dinner and end the day in a relaxing way. 'I'm always looking forward to that', he said laughing. This experience, shared by a service-user during a public discussion, links to the argument present throughout the analysis of the recovery assemblage, that the connections made within the group are not solely, potentially not even primarily, based on suffering. They equally build on desires of becomings, on hopes and aspirations for a future that has not yet become and on aspects of sociality that go beyond the consumption (or not) of substances. Most importantly, they are also vital for the present of people in recovery and the connections between them that take place inside and outside the recovery space, whether these connections are made over sharing food and laughter, or through sharing trauma and intense rehearsals. Finally, it is these diverse connections – processes like 'turning up' and 'checking-in', the generation of safety, hope and boundaries, and the socialities emerging in the recovery and creative groups, in other words the material, affective and social recovery assemblage – that unblock and carry the service-users' flows of desire beyond the space of recovery.

However, it needs to be acknowledged that connections between people in recovery and other socialities, discussed above, are mediated by the recovery assemblage; through this mediation the social becomes an extension of the recovery space, where service-users can make new connections while remaining in a protective, safe and caring framework. In what follows, I explore how participants from Athens view the social environment in which they are expected to 'reintegrate' after their disengagement from 18 ano. I do so focusing on the visual material produced during our photography walks, the conversations that emerged from the pictures, and the responses of the service-users when asked if they would like 18 ano to be different in any way.

Figure 6.4 was taken by one of the service-users during a photography walk at the area of Kypseli. Later on, when we were discussing the photographs in the group, the photographer said:

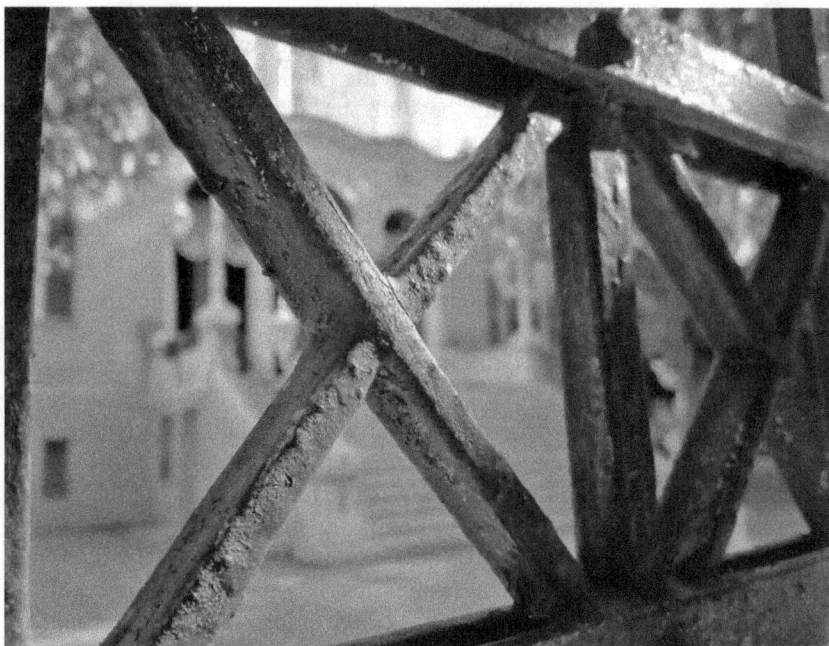

Figure 6.4 The church, Athens.

*That's a church at the back. This touches lot of different sides of mine ...
how they [formal institutions] create this feeling, disappointment that is,
unfairness and pretentiousness, the pretended interest ... everything is rusty
[building an allegory between the rusty barriers of the photograph and the
institutions], like they don't exist, I don't even see them.*

This conversation took place in March 2017, approximately eight years since
the beginning of the debt crisis of 2009, which led to an 'overwhelming pessimism about the economic and political situation in the country, matched
with almost unanimous disapproval of leading political and institutional fig-
ures for their responsibility in bringing the country to the verge of bankruptcy'
(Triandafyllidou, Gropas and Kouki, 2013: 7). This pessimism that grew
during the years of the crisis was the outburst of the question of 'where do we
belong?' which has always been quintessential for the national collective consciousness, since the creation of the Greek state in the 19th century (ibid.: 9).
Especially during its recent, post-1974 (post-dictatorship) history, the Greek
state has been defined by a tension between tradition and modernity known as
'cultural dualism' a term deployed to describe the contradictions that emerged
through the encounter of the Ottoman rule with the European Enlightenment
(between East and West) (ibid: 2–4). Figure 6.4 visualises this tension by
problematising the role of the Orthodox church – an institution that remains
'constitutionally sheltered and retains its stronghold on the country's civic and,
on occasion, political life' (ibid.: 4) – and by rejecting the distinction between
'traditional' and 'modern' Westernised institutions since *'everything is rusty,
like they don't exist, I don't even see them'*. While in other national contexts –
and recovery approaches – tensions associated with the political and cultural
domination of institutions like the church extend to the ways that recovery is
practised (Zigon, 2011), 18 ano has resisted the replication of dominant power
structures through the practice of recovery. Through this resistance, the juxtaposition between the social assemblage of recovery and the social assemblages
dominated by authoritative institutions becomes highly visible and affective.

In Figure 6.5 and the commentary that follows, the photographer expresses
this same tension between tradition and modernity, not through the rejection
of the institution but through his identification with non-human components
that constitute the 'Athenian' assemblage.

*An image of Athens, double standards, luxuries and modernisation and
Europe, look at this for example. There are two buildings, relatively new,
and I very often feel like [I am] the one in the middle, that I'm under
pressure from all directions and that I need renovation and that's what I'm
called to do.*

Here, the service-user, identifying with the collective consciousness of
ambiguity between the past and the future, acknowledges that he needs

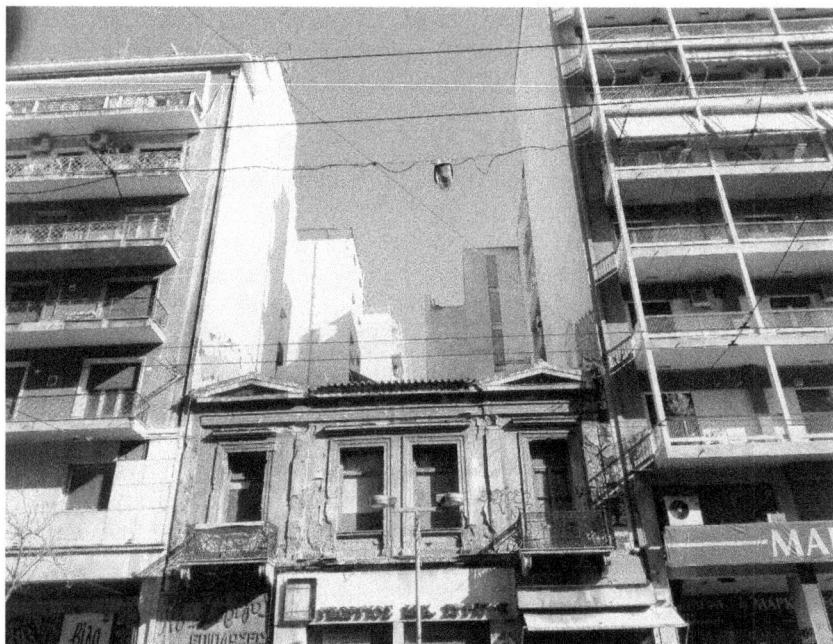

Figure 6.5 Renovation, Athens.

'renovation'. Whilst in the recovery assemblage this process of 'renovation' was experienced as a collective desire of becoming-other, when positioned in the Athenian public space it turns into the outcome of being '*under pressure from all directions*'. The desire of becoming-other and the deterritorialisations that became possible through the affective and caring practices produced in the recovery assemblage, run the risk of being reterritorialised when trying to connect with other assemblages, perceived as oppressive and hostile. This problematic transition is also reflected on the way boundaries are understood, inside and outside the recovery assemblage:

> *I took this picture [figure 6.6] thinking of reality today. You try to start something new, something specific, you can't within this logic of restriction and lack of freedom of movement. In general I have an issue with restrictions. I'm not talking about power issues that go deeper, I'm talking about simple things that work for me in a reactionary way. If you tell me 'don't do that', that's very different than explaining to me that if I do that [this will happen]. The 'no's', the 'don'ts' the 'mustn't, the 'musts' that's all very hard for me.*

When exploring the affective recovery assemblage, the process of establishing boundaries was discussed as a practice of care that does not aim to restrict the

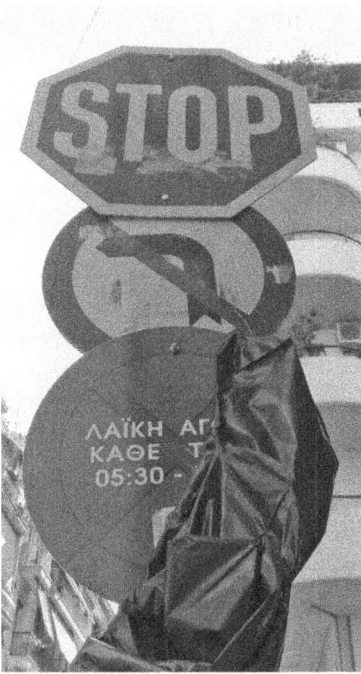

Figure 6.6 Stop, Athens.

'freedom of movement' of service-users. Conversely, the aim is the enhance-ment of a body's capacity to act through the enablement of connections that take into consideration the collective and individual needs of all actors involved. Figure 6.6 however and the commentary that follows it, demon-strate that the constraints that accompany *'reality today'* are not there to enhance but to block a body's capacity to act. The desire of becoming-other, *'to start something new'* is blocked by *'this logic of restriction and lack of freedom of movement'*. The boundaries of the recovery assemblage are indir-ectly compared to the restrictions that one has to confront in other social assemblages. In recovery, the boundaries and constraints can be explained and negotiated as they are not imposed from above but develop organic-ally and with the purpose of enabling the connections produced within the recovery assemblage. However, the imposing 'STOP' sign photographed from below is experienced as a symbol of restrictions that are put in place to regu-late and control; to block connections, rather than to enhance them.

These contradictory experiences of boundaries and constraints as enhancements of connections when negotiated and developed organic-ally, and as obstacles of one's becoming-other when imposed by dominant forces and institutions, resonate with empirical data produced by studies exploring recovery from mental illness through the deployment of the Deleuzo–Guattarian assemblage. Price-Robertson, Manderson and Duff (2017), in their analysis of the affective power of the family assemblage in recovery from mental illness, account for Felix's, one of their participants, shifting experience of boundaries and constraints. While Felix's identity was for many years 'cohered around defiance of the authorities in his life' (Price-Robertson, Manderson and Duff, 2017: 420), his subsequent becoming with the family assemblage shifted his perception of himself from a body disciplined and oppressed by the medical apparatus, to a body willing to abide with certain boundaries and constraints in order to maintain the ties that enhance its wellbeing. This analysis also reflects McLeod's understanding of boundaries and limits placed on the processes of transformation as practices that 'increase the affective intensity of life in a manageable way. These limits are also productive in spurring the production of assemblages with different kinds of capacities' (McLeod, 2017: 99). Such examples from the recovery (from mental health and drugs) assemblage empirically account for the reterritorialising force of boundaries and constraints when these are imposed from outside, and conversely, their ability to enhance a body's power of acting when emerging from connections produced within the assemblage.

Back to the Athenian social assemblage, the assemblages service-users will have to eventually become part of, are perceived as hostile, restrictive and oppressive when not mediated by the recovery assemblage. This perception is not arbitrarily formed, and does not only concern people in recovery, but draws on a national collective consciousness that cannot find its place between the traditions that draw from the East and the call for modernisation coming from the West. The understanding of the institutions that form the Greek state as hostile and restrictive – symbolically presented in the photographs of the Athenian public space – is further induced by the austerity measures taken, presented as necessary in order to overcome the financial crisis, further restricting the options of those called to 'reintegrate' in this particular social reality.

This contradiction between the inside and outside of the recovery assemblage is regarded by some of the service-users as problematic; the recovery assemblage becomes a non-realistically protective space that does not prepare them for the assemblages they will have to become part of following their disengagement from the recovery service:

> If you want my opinion, one thing that I don't like about 18 [ano] is that it doesn't present realistically the 'outside'. The fact that in 18 [ano] we all love each other, we're all next to each other, when leaving [you realise that] it's an illusion and that's a shock to the system … It's not the same. There's solidarity and comradeship but only for as long as you're in 18 [ano].

These contradictions, fears and insecurities linked to the current Greek social reality, have led to a call by the service-users for a longer-lasting protective and caring environment, an extended period of time for them to stay in-between the recovery assemblage and other socialities:

> *I'd like it if it [the recovery programme] didn't end here. I feel that it'll end and I'm gonna miss everything good that I've created and I feel a bit insecure ... I'd like it if there was one more stage, of a looser form, somehow to continue. I don't know, I like all this and I don't want it to end.*

The call of the service-user above, for an 'extension' of the recovery time, echoes the historical and current particularities of the Greek society that block the transition of the recovering body from the recovery assemblage to other socialities. Within the recovery assemblage, the financial crisis has been dealt with by strengthening a shared subjectivity and, through art groups and other activities this has been extended to other social assemblages. However, when the recovery assemblage ceases operating as a mediator for service-users between the inside and outside, then the fear to confront social reality prevails, and leads to a call for the recovery assemblage to remain present, even in a *'looser form'*. In what follows I examine the case of Liverpool, and how Genie's social recovery assemblage extends to the city of Liverpool's social assemblage through participation and engagement with creative aspects of the city.

Liverpool

As stated on Genie's website, a significant part of the organisation's vision is the promotion of social inclusion through increasing participation in the creative arts (www.genieinthegutter.co.uk/). Drawing on the visual material produced by Genie's service-users, I explore how social inclusion happens in practice through the creative activities of Genie. I do so mobilising Duff's (2011) concept of enabling places, deployed to demonstrate the relationship between social inclusion and recovery from primary health problems:

> *Places are rarely settled and their coordinates are never fixed. They are forever mobilised, transformed and reproduced in the dynamic force of inhabiting place. To conceive of an ecology of enabling places is to emphasise this material and relational production of place ... enabling places are made rather than merely discovered.*
>
> (Duff, 2011: 155)

The visual material produced by Genie's service-users and the descriptions that accompany them, reveal the array of connections made possible through the artistic practices taking place within and beyond the recovery space.

Through these encounters enabling places are made, enhancing a body's capacity to act. Within this framework, artistic practice is not simply discussed as a form of 'expression', but as *a force of connection* between the social recovery assemblage and the social assemblages extending beyond it. According to Deleuze and Guattari, art causes 'increasingly decoded and deterritorialized flows to circulate in the socius, flows that are perceptible to everyone, which force the social axiomatic to grow ever more complicated, to become more saturated' (Deleuze and Guattari, 1977: 379). However, the connection of the recovery body with other social assemblages is not unconditionally 'good'. Memories of exclusion and the embodiment of self-blame often accompany the becomings of people in recovery, rendering their connection with other assemblages complicated, especially when these are not mediated by the recovery assemblage. The question that arises through the engagement of Genie's service-users with artistic practices, is whether this engagement can challenge the exclusions that accompany drug using bodies, and transform socialities, opening them up to the inclusion of all bodies, rather than just the 'recovered' ones.

I took a picture of the art gallery because we'd just been there and it's just an example of some of the stuff I'd done at Genie that I wouldn't normally do like before I came to Genie, I wouldn't have gone to art galleries or museums really to look at exhibitions and stuff like that. If you're just

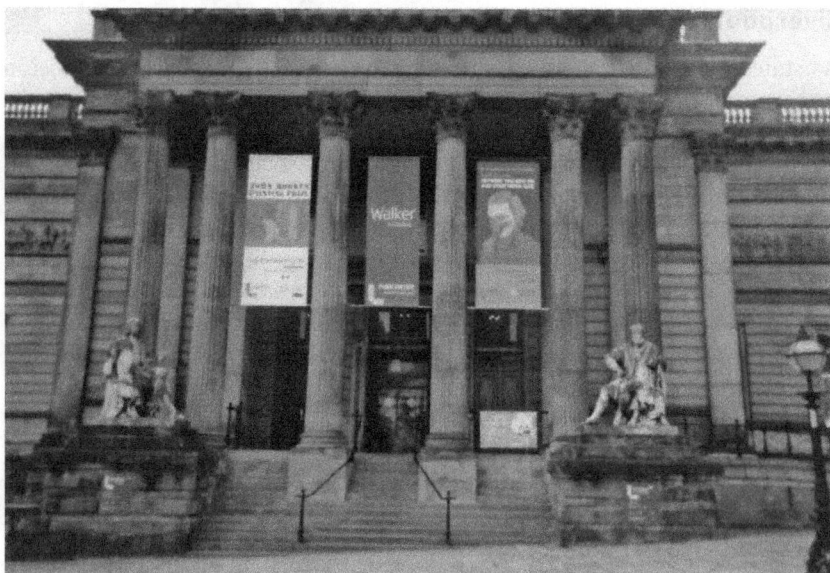

Figure 6.7 The Gallery, Liverpool.

wandering around, some sort of pointless drunk and then you only get to see the outside of buildings. I do actually appreciate the architecture and that but you always feel like you're barred and you're not allowed in or something, like you go past a nice pub but you can't go in there [laughs] or a nice building or a nice hotel, you know, you're not going to stay there, or a nice, a sort of like upmarket shop or something, you know you're not going to go in there to buy stuff and that. So there's that sense of exclusion. So it's like the doorways are a metaphor, like you can go in like you know, I think because a lot of it's just your own mindset isn't it? You've convinced yourself you don't belong, so you stay outside of everything! But it's nice to have people to like encourage you to sort of take part I suppose on the indoor culture side of things! Because when I first came here, you know it was nice to go to other places where other things are happening ... or when we were going to the cathedral to play the drums outside and stuff like that, to go somewhere and get inside and get involved.

The above is an account of the *making* of an enabling place, the connections that render its becoming possible and the new encounters that derive from it. The service-user describes the visit to the gallery as a new experience that became possible through his engagement with Genie, providing an example of how the recovery assemblage extends to other assemblages and generates affective encounters that enable participation in *'the indoor culture side of things'*. Being 'outside' is symbolically talked about as a space of exclusion. The gallery space becomes an enabling place due to the way that it is experienced; a space that becomes accessible with others, with people that *'encourage you to take part'*. Another aspect of the above narrative to be taken into consideration is the photographer's embodiment of self-blame for his past exclusion from institutions like art galleries. As a *'pointless drunk wandering around ... you always feel like you're barred and you're not allowed in or something'*. Rather than criticising the institution for the exclusions that it reproduces, the responsibility shifts to the excluded: *'I think because a lot of it's just your own mindset isn't it? You've convinced yourself you don't belong, so you stay outside of everything!'* Following this line of thought, the doorways of the buildings work as a metaphor, separating those who 'belong' from those who *convince themselves* they *'don't belong'*. The recovery assemblage, extending to other institutions and socialities renders the 'inside' possible, as well as desired (*it was nice to go to other places where other things are happening*); but the internalisation of the exclusions that using bodies suffer, persists. The transition from a using to a recovering body, from the 'outside' to the 'inside', is ongoing and under negotiation, when permission to gain access is asked:

Well I have to press the button and say who I am, but they let me in though, when I've said who I am, which is like, still come to terms with that, it's me [laughs] can I come in, are you sure, I just said it's me, like, are you

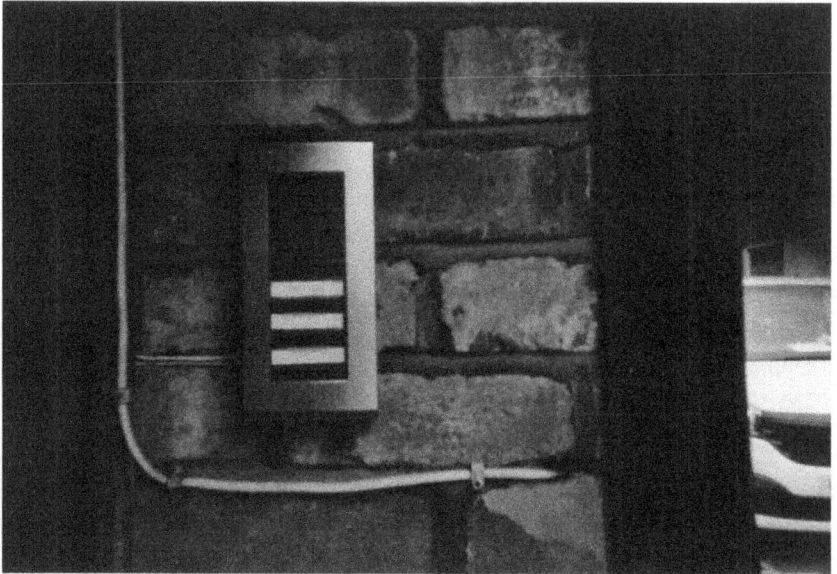

Figure 6.8 The Buzzer, Liverpool.

> *absolutely sure?! [laughs] But yeah … Well I suppose it's a symbol of the
> fact I'm connected at least.*

The doorways of the previous picture are now replaced by the buzzer, the
'gatekeeper' of one of the creative services the service-user is engaged with,
standing in-between the 'inside' and the 'outside'. The narrator still tries to
'*come to terms with*' the fact that it is by stating who he is that access is granted.
In his words, the door that opens when he says his name is '*a symbol of the
fact I'm connected*'. This 'surprise' that comes with one's inclusion is described
by one of Genie's workers as a 'challenge' for those used to being excluded:

> *I think he [one of Genie's service-users] can't believe that he's still accessing
> us and hasn't been excluded, because he gets excluded everywhere he goes.
> I think that for him has been his biggest challenge in accepting that, that
> regardless of his behaviour, we'll still work with it!*

In these visual and oral narratives, the opening doors are symbols of
connections, and the ones that remain shut are symbols of disconnection
and isolation. When mediated by the recovery assemblage, connections with
other social assemblages become possible, while the drug using, individual
body remains 'outside', embodying systems that render it accountable for

its isolation. This reflects the previous discussion about the Athenian social space: extending to other socialities with the recovery assemblage produced a dynamic interaction, transformative of the socialities the recovery assemblage was extending to. Conversely, when the recovering body was imagining its presence in the social outside the recovery assemblage, public spaces were perceived as hostile and threatening. These accounts emphasise the significance of the connections produced inside the recovery assemblage, and how these enhance a body's capacity to act. At the same time, they problematise long-standing questions of inclusion and exclusion that the recovering body experiences in its attempt to extend to other assemblages. I now shift my focus from the public to the private space of service-users, to explore how it is transformed through the connections produced in the recovery assemblage.

> *That's an oil painting I did because I felt inspired, because I was doing the art classes here [Genie] and ... I'd found a canvas and I'd found a bag full of different paints and art materials and stuff, and some of it was oil paints and thought it would be interesting to do an oil painting because I'd never done an oil painting, I'd done all sorts of other types of art but I hadn't done an oil painting. So one day when I just felt like it, I just sat down and did it, because I had the canvas and I had the oil paints so I thought why not, so I did it! I was pretty pleased with the results!*

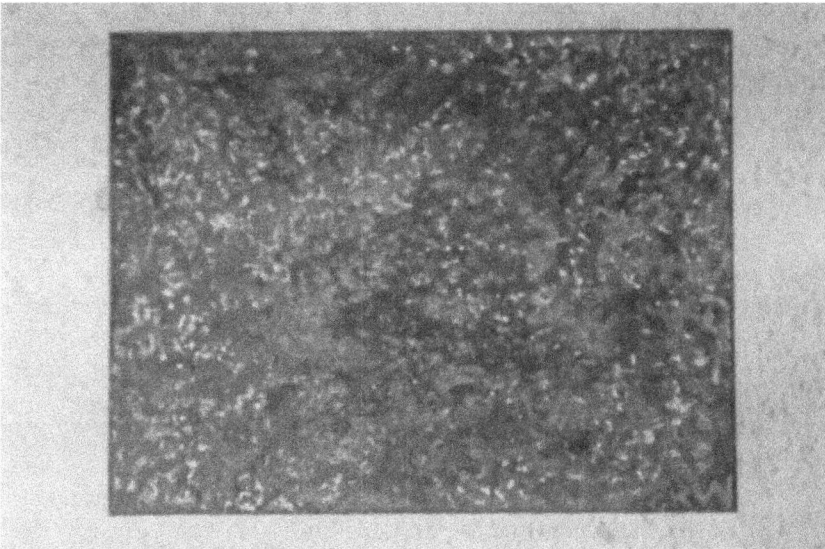

Figure 6.9 The oil painting, Liverpool.

The oil painting depicted in Figure 6.9 is the outcome of an encounter between the 'inside' and the 'outside'. The 'inspiration' comes from the creative practices taking place within the recovery assemblage, while the materials are found and collected 'outside'. This encounter produces an oil painting in the private space of the service-user. Following the route of these various encounters opens up the way for a wider understanding of 'enabling places', as places that are not only produced on the sites where the encounters take place but extend beyond them and include social as well as private places. In the description above, the private place becomes an enabling one when the desire continues to flow beyond the recovery assemblage, actively looking for encounters that enhance a body's capacity to act. The art classes at Genie generate a desire, an *inspiration*, to use the words of the service-user that extends to other places, like the street, where the materials for the production of the oil painting are found, and eventually to the private space, where the painting is produced. While under different circumstances these found watercolours might not have been regarded as an opportunity for creative practice, the narrator allows himself to be affected by this random encounter, extending it to his private space where the art work is produced.

It has been discussed how creative practices in the recovery assemblage and their extension to other socialities enhance the inclusion of bodies in spaces from where they have been excluded in the past, and enhance their desire for connection through creativity. At the same time, the narrations of these encounters render visible the exclusions of the past, and potentially the future, when the connection with the recovery assemblage will not be possible. The following photograph and account that accompanies it, provides a final example of how all these different layers of connections – personal and shared experiences and places – come together when creative, recovery practices extend to the social, linking past memories with present practices.

> That's the Everyman,[4] a shot of the Everyman from outside and, I mean on the face of it, it's just showing all different types of people, so I was thinking of it as a metaphor for like there's all different types of recovery and things that you need to recover from and stuff like that. But also, my mother's wake was actually held in the Everyman. And also I had a big photo of myself up in the Everyman, because they did a project, it was linked to Genie and a few Genie clients had like huge big blow-up photos of themselves, they were all lined up inside the Everyman and it was part of some project, I'm not exactly sure which. But that was quite a proud moment, because you know a big blow-up photo of yourself somewhere in, as prominent as the Everyman foyer are sort of thing it was in. And I went to see it, and yeah, it was quite good. But yeah, so there's that link.

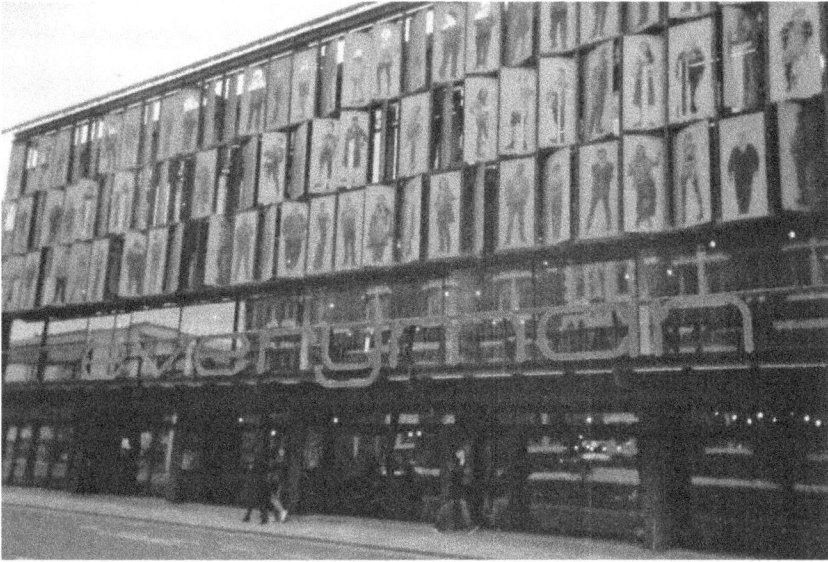

Figure 6.10 Everyman, Liverpool.

In this description the first connection to be accounted for is the one between the '*different types of people*' shown outside the Everyman, and how this image works as a metaphor for '*all different types of recovery and things that you need to recover from*'. This connection does not only extend the recovery assemblage beyond the recovery space, but also challenges stereotypical representations of the isolated and dehumanised addict (Fitzgerald, 2015). In the narrations accompanying the photographs discussed earlier, the exclusion of the drug using body was normalised. Instead, here the recovering body does not stand in isolation, nor in connection only with other human components of the recovery assemblage, but in connection with all '*different types of people*', a metaphor in the photographer's analysis of his picture for '*all different types of recovery*'. The narration then moves on from the 'outside' to the interior of the Everyman Theatre, where the connections briefly extend to the service-user's personal life prior to his engagement with recovery (*my mother's wake was actually held in the Everyman*), before providing another link between the '*different types of people*' shown at the front of the building and the presence of the recovering subject beyond the recovery space (*also I had a big photo of myself up in the Everyman, because they did a project, it was linked to Genie*). The Everyman becomes thus a place that enables the connection of the recovery assemblage with the social, the connection between past and new experiences, and the inclusion of the recovering body in the social space.

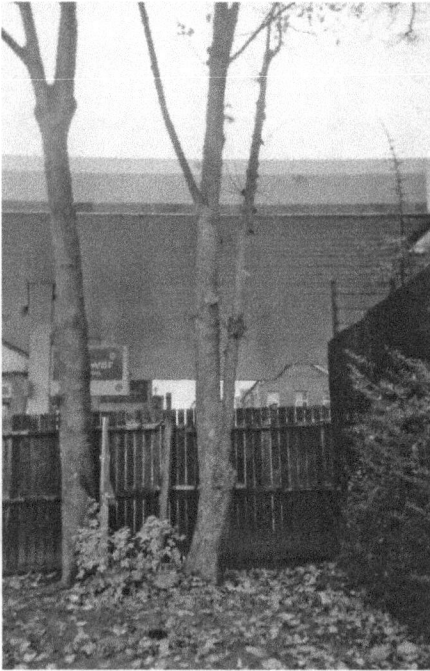

Figure 6.11 Supported accommodation, Liverpool.

I now return to how private spaces are experienced, how the potentials of these assemblages are expanded through the encounter with the recovery assemblage, but also how they are blocked by forces of reterritorialisation. The following presentation of a service-user's place of residence comes to show that the enablement of encounters by the recovery assemblage is considered essential in order to stay connected with the 'outside' and avoid isolation.

Photographer: Oh that's outside, that's my garden, well part of the garden. It's called sheltered accommodation. I've lived in all kinds of accommodations you know and you need somewhere that you feel safe and secure in you know. But they're not, there's thirty seven residents, well they say there's thirty seven residents but I only know about six of them and I've been there two years, six out of thirty seven!

Interviewer: Where are the rest of them?

Photographer: I think they're just becoming cabbages in their rooms you know, neglected ... it's [the accommodation] not conducted to your mental health or your well, or your natural health. They have no activities, you know?

I'm getting very lazy you know mentally. Because I don't have any stimula-
tion, you see what I mean? That's the problem. That's why I come here [to
Genie], to get some stimulation.

The conversation above is telling of not only the role of the recovery assemblage in making enabling spaces but also in maintaining these connections.
Although each event of social connection contributes to the growth and
'becoming well' of the recovering body, and the enhancement of the
assemblage's power of acting (Duff, 2014a: 113), it is also essential that we
take seriously the everyday lives of the recovering bodies, inside, as well as
outside the recovery assemblage. The encounter with the recovery assemblage
produces the desire to extend the possible connections to other assemblages,
like the sheltered accommodation discussed above. However, these places
are '*not conducted to your mental health, or your natural health*', they are
not conducted to enhance connections, rendering the return to the recovery
assemblage necessary, for the desire of becoming connected to flow.

Although transitionality and temporality are foundational characteristics
of the recovery assemblage, the visual and oral accounts of service-users
from both Liverpool and Athens call for an extension, not necessarily of the
recovering practices as such, but of the caring practices and the connections
and encounters that become possible through the recovery assemblage. This
need, produces becoming well as an ongoing process without an end point;
it requires constant work, a nurturing and expansion of the connections
established (McLeod, 2017). A clear distinction however needs to be made
between a call for a prolonged provision of care, and a medicalised discourse
that understands addiction as a chronic, relapsing disease of the brain, leading
to the pathologisation of drug use and the stigmatisation of (recovering) drug
users as chronically ill individuals, eternally dependent on services.

When facilitating one of the recovery groups at Genie, I asked the service-
users if, according to them, there is an end date to the recovery process. While
a couple of them stated that recovery was for them a bridge between addiction
and their future plans, and therefore did have an end date, the majority of the
group talked about recovery as 'a way of being'. As has been the case with
various other arguments made throughout the previous chapters, here as well
it is not the substance positioned as the focus of attention. When members of
the group were asked to elaborate what recovery as a 'way of being' means to
them, they did not talk about relapses, substitutes and substances, but of the
need to *maintain the connections* produced within the recovery assemblage. For
some of them this could take the form of volunteering for a service, becoming
sponsors in AA and NA meetings, or just permanently attending structured
recovery groups a couple of times per week. Their response to my question
challenges medicalised approaches, which consider recovery's only purpose
to be the separation of the body from the substance. Conversely, it has been
argued and demonstrated through the oral and visual data produced that the

aim of the recovery process is not to block and separate, but to connect and enable encounters that enhance a body's capacity to act. Through the accounts of service-users it has become apparent that recovery is not about *not doing* – not using drugs for example – but about *doing and engaging*, finding an active way of being that maintains the connections that enhance a body's power of acting. This way of thinking and experiencing recovery challenges the construction of the autonomous 'recovered' individual, blameable when not able to connect with other assemblages.

In what follows, I further explore this desire to 'stay connected' through the accounts of service-users when asked how they imagine or desire their lives to be after recovery. This is juxtaposed to their fears associated with being 'outside' the recovery assemblage, and with recovery as it is produced through policymaking. I argue that while service-users desire the deterritorialisation of the new becomings produced in the recovery assemblage, dominant neoliberal practices operate as reterritorialising forces that block these new becomings. I extend this line of thought to discuss how policymaking practices block the provision of care that enhances the recovering body's capacity to act, by diminishing the freedom of service-workers to work together *with* service-users towards the production of new, desired becomings.

Finally, my aim is to imagine how policymaking can be done otherwise. My intention is to challenge the common tendency of asking how a better drug policy can lead to the provision of better recovery. Instead, I shift the question in order to ask *how we can enable the recovery assemblage to unconditionally provide the practices of care that are in place already*. How can policy enhance those practices without trying to regulate them? How can we better enable the recovery assemblage to transform the assemblages it comes into contact with? How can we deterritorialise the recovery assemblage?

Notes

1　Service-users are excluded from the group activities but not from the programme overall. They still get to meet their therapists and after a certain period of time they re-enter the group activities.
2　Andreas Loverdos was the Minister of Health from September 2010 until May 2012.
3　For an overview of the events and occupation of ERT see Guardian (2013) www.theguardian.com/world/2013/jun/11/state-broadcaster-ert-shut-down-greece and Goat (2015) www.opendemocracy.net/en/can-europe-make-it/greeces-two-year-blackout-static-suicide-and-new-selfmanagement-model/
4　Theatre and cultural centre located in the city of Liverpool.

Chapter 7

Beyond the recovery assemblage

Chapter 5 focused on the service-users' desire of becoming-other, and on how this desire was invested in drug use, until it became blocked. I then moved on to the analysis of the recovery assemblage, closely following the process of becoming a service-user. I argued that in recovery, the flows of desire are becoming unblocked through three articulations: the material, affective and social recovery assemblage, showing how practices of care pave the way for the deterritorialisation of flows of desire and enable novel connections, thus, enhancing a body's capacity to act.

I now discuss the shape and form that these deterritorialisations take in the hopes and aspirations of service-users for a future yet to become. My aim is to provide an alternative approach to the existing literature on recovery that focuses on a critique of the neoliberal political rationality produced within the recovery assemblage (Fomiatti, Moore and Fraser, 2019). The recovery assemblage can be approached as a space of resistance, rather than subordination to this neoliberal political rationality, and my critique focuses on the forces and institutions that operate *outside* it and block the deterritorialisations becoming within the recovery space. Staying with the lines of flight emerging from the recovery assemblage, constitutes a different way of thinking about policy, a careful way that aims at the establishment of policy as a force whose role is to enable, rather than to block the deterritorilisations that become possible through the practices of care that organically emerge in recovery.

> *We're not angels and the guys [service-users] aren't angels either and we don't want them to become angels, we're not interested in that ... This is a recovery programme, not an angels' construction programme.*

This statement, made by one of 18 ano's art therapists, challenges the view that the aim of recovery is to produce a desire for normalisation (Nettleton, Neale and Pickering, 2013), and is in line with previous accounts of workers from both services when discussing the affective flows that become possible within the recovery assemblage. Creating an enabling (Duff, 2011),

DOI: 10.4324/9781003165613-8

caring space and focusing on acknowledging the service-users' desires rather than imposing norms on them, have been fundamental components of the connections produced in the recovery assemblage. The statement above as well as the accounts that follow are responses to my questions concerning the service-users' lives after the recovery process has been completed. The desire of becoming-other, is now trying to extend to other assemblages. Employment, motherhood and having a routine are negotiated by service-users and workers as assemblages that have to be shaped and transformed in order to support the desire of becoming-well. Yet, this desire clashes with neoliberal perceptions of worthiness and functionality. I conclude that it is this exact battle that policy's role is to resolve, shifting from a focus on specific recommendations that prioritise one treatment approach over another, and the invention of tools for the 'measurement' of outcomes, to a practice that allows for the organically produced practices of care to grow, and supports the enhancement of the recovering body's capacity to act within and beyond the recovery assemblage.

Becoming content, becoming connected

> I've just started looking for a job and I find it difficult already. There are people that were never using [drugs] and yet they're stressed about picking up the phone, going to interviews, I'm very stressed about it but I'm going to make it … I also think it's very important to have things that make you happy and content because we're all bored of routine … A circle is closing but the therapy continues in a different way.

> I'm looking very much into theatre, the theatre game for example could include lots of the things I do. I'll take some acting and dramatherapy lessons to get in touch with the field outside 18 [ano], to see if this can really give me what I need. And the job I have now, I work as a kitchen porter, I'm definitely going to keep it for a while.

In these accounts, there is a tension between 'having a job' and 'becoming content'. While becoming employed is discussed as something that needs to be done, even if it is a source of stress ('I'm very stressed about it but I'm going to make it', 'I'm definitely going to keep [my job] for a while'), the desire lies elsewhere. In the first narrative it is *other* things that can make one happy and content, and these need to be explored, as part of a therapeutic process that continues beyond the recovery assemblage *in a different way*. In the second account, while having a job (*for a while*) is essential, it is a creative practice ('*I'm looking very much into theatre*') that can potentially *include lots of the things* that the narrator does and *give her what she needs*. In other words, becoming content, meaning here the emotional fulfilment that derives from one's daily practices, is achieved through the exploration of activities that are desired, rather than through the establishment of a working routine, which in many cases is presented as the 'antidote' to the 'chaotic lifestyle' associated with addiction (Sumnall and Brotherhood, 2012; Perkins, 2008; Spencer et al., 2008; Neale and Kemp, 2009).

However, even when work is desired in one's everyday life, the drive for this desire is the connections and encounters made possible within a working environment. Once more, 'having a job' is to be negotiated and thought about according to one's needs:

> *I've trained as a chef but I don't think that I'll choose to continue with that because of the isolation and alienation due to the working hours. When everyone rests I have to work and I don't see how this would be helpful for my recovery, if I'm isolated from the people around me. I've worked as a manager in a restaurant and the only target is to take the clients' money and make them come back, I don't think that works for me ... Ideally I'd like to open a restaurant and work with ex drug users. I'd like to open such a space that operates with the standards of a therapeutic space, not like a business. Of course it'd have to meet certain criteria and the competition out there, but would be run collectively and there would be solidarity amongst the workers.*

> *I'd like to have a job that I enjoy doing, achieving that's not that easy. Take the film-making course I'm doing at the moment, I mean it's nice to have dreams and everything like you know, but you've got to be practical haven't you? So I'd love to be a world class writer/director or superstar actor or something but as far as that course is concerned, that's key as being realistic as well. I think I'd be good at lighting say for example, because we've done quite a lot of the technical stuff and I seem to have a flare for that. So that would be good, if I could do something like that, where you know I'm working in an environment that's interesting, I'm doing something that's interesting, I'm surrounded by interesting people, then I'd look forward to going to work you know, it would be fun.*

These two narratives provide a way of thinking about employment that positions wellbeing and the enablement of meaningful connections as the focus of attention. In the first account, the desire to maintain abstinence from drugs is prioritised over the working skills that the service-user already holds ('*I don't think that I'll choose to continue with that*'). The process of getting a job is not discussed with regards to what is easily achievable, but in relation to the desires that derive from the values the service-user wants to apply in his everyday encounters ('*I'd like to open such a space that operates with the standards of a therapeutic space, not like a business*'). Accordingly, in the second account, the focus is on finding the right balance between desirable and realistic work options ('*it's nice to have dreams and everything like you know, but you've got to be practical haven't you?*'). Potential job options are identified following a frame of thought that reflects self-awareness of the skills that can be obtained ('*I seem to have a flare for that*') as well as of the desired connections. This understanding of work as an assemblage that needs to address one's desires and provide more than wages, is also reflected on the therapeutic framework of 18 ano, as explained by one of the programme's social workers:

> *Work constitutes an important part of the therapy process, but not a compulsory one, because through work [service-users] will not only cover basic needs. They will also cover social needs. They will relate with their employer, their colleagues, their clients. They will cover emotional needs, recognition, the ability to set targets and achieve them, trust, co-existence with other people … working doesn't mean having a job. [Work] offers you the opportunity to grow, to get to know yourself, your limits … Work is very important when not done in an opportunistic way, but with programming. What do I want to do? What skills do I need? How can I develop them?*

The work-related desires of service-users and the way work is talked about and negotiated within the recovery assemblage are not in harmony with neoliberal systems of thought where 'having a job' is identified as the primary factor for the measurement of a person's value. Enhancing a body's capacity to act should not be associated with a never-ending increase of demands, but with the ability to also acknowledge and accept a body's limitations. As accurately put by Genie's keyworker, at some point, we have to say 'that's enough':

> *That's amazing and that's enough. Stop making demands and accept that that's the way it is because I absolutely believe everyone is capable of giving something back but in their own way and in their own time, and it doesn't always got to be through taxes.*

As emphasised by both services in Liverpool and Athens, 'getting a job' has to be acknowledged as a time-consuming process that needs to be done carefully in order to keep service-users safe:

> *And you know it sounds like a long time, but actually if you think about all the skills you need to develop in that time and how stressful work is anyway for most of us, and how many people probably regularly drink to cope with work and how that can easily become an issue … I think it's ignorant of the Government to think that once you remove a substance someone's, oh OK they're back to work, they've got normal life again, because if that was the case, they wouldn't be misusing the substance to the point of addiction, because they wouldn't need to.*

Based on Genie's manager's account above, becoming employed does not only need to be considered as a potential risk for people *after* they disengage from recovery, but it also might be associated with the reasons they started using at first place. These are all aspects that are not taken into consideration by drug policies that unconditionally link employability with recovery (e.g. HM Government, 2010 and 2017), without addressing the risks associated with it. While service-users express the desire for a deterritorialised perception of employability that prioritises connections, neoliberal practices push for the reterritorialisation of this desire by producing employability as an unconditional responsibility of the recovering subject.

I now provide another example of deterritorialisation, rendered possible through encounters produced in the recovery assemblage. Although gender has not been addressed, as this would require more time and space than is available to properly elaborate on this issue, the following is a response of 18 ano's children's' psychologist when asked if, during the recovery process, the aim is to reconnect the mothers with their children. The aim here is not to discuss motherhood as such, but to further expand on the argument that through the recovery assemblage new connections become possible, connections that go beyond prefabricated perceptions of aspects that define sociality, including employability and motherhood.

The priority is to see the characteristics of all the people involved [in the upbringing of a child], the mother, the child, other relatives, the social and financial background and to shape the best possible development, appropriate for all. This can take various different shapes. We don't ask for the mother to be the primary carer for her child, if this doesn't really represent the mother, her needs, her desires and her capacities. If this [to become the primary carer] is articulated by the mother then the programme will support it 100%. If things though are not exactly like that, and through her therapy process [the mother] sees things about herself and lets herself free to detect her desires and her strengths, then it is a challenge indeed to find a way to support the mother and the child so that they both have positive experiences of each other, without looking for prefabricated solutions. To be more specific, a child might grow up at the house of its grandparents if this is wanted by everyone, and the mother can have a very good, consistent relationship with it. There have been many such stories. Each mother and child have written their own story. The same mother with more than one children might have a different story with each one of them. The older child for example might stay under the grandparents' care ... while the second child might be raised by her, potentially together with a partner that might be the father of the child or not. We can't know any of this in advance and we can't operate based on our own standards because we don't know where these come from ... All we care about is for the child to have its needs met. If a mother develops her mental maturity that much, that she can understand what her child's needs are and can say I'm not in a position to cover these needs but I can activate this and that mechanism, then for us that's a success.

Just like employability was negotiated in the recovery assemblage in a fashion that prioritised the desires of service-users, becoming a mother is discussed as a process that can take various different forms, covering the needs of everyone involved. Going beyond *'prefabricated solutions'* is a key phrase that accurately summarises the practices of care becoming in the recovery assemblage. It is through these novel connections and encounters that deterritorialisation becomes possible and, most importantly, desired. What is at stake here is how policymaking and the expectations that it (re)produces attempt to reterritorialise the lines of flight that extend beyond the recovery assemblage. Employment, when perceived as a timely process of making connections and exploring desires, clashes with neoliberal systems of thought. Accordingly, becoming a mother, developing a consistent and meaningful relationship with one's child outside existing family models, clashes with prefabricated perceptions of maternal love. In what follows I draw on the same argument, by demonstrating how becoming content and connected does not only relate to having an occupation, whether this takes the form of a job or of the engagement with other activities, but also through becoming one-self and developing the ability to enjoy 'small things':

In the past I thought that something extraordinary had to happen [in order to be happy]. Now it's my everyday life [that makes me happy], the fact that I can sleep, really sleep. And I'm happy with small things, I'm happy without carrying a burden all the time.

I've managed to be happy with simple things. While in the past something massive had to happen for me to say that I'm good. Even with the coffee that I'm making in the morning, opening the window, for me it's very important … [When I look at myself] I see a human being, I see a woman, not an exhausted girl … The choices, the love, the care, the patience to do things, to not be in a rush all the time, for me that's life.

In the above, both participants narrate how becoming happy in the past, was only possible through *'extraordinary'* and *'massive'* events. They put emphasis on their current ability to enjoy *'small things'*, to enjoy *'everyday life'* without being in a rush. Finally, becoming content and connected is also associated with the ability to be one-self:

Just be my best, just be myself and be my best, do the best I can and hopefully like you know that's good enough, if it's not then so be it. You know but as long as I'm happy within myself and everything, or content, and I like myself [laughs], that will do me, it really will.

The analysis of such empirical accounts that refer to everyday life, small things, routines and mundane tasks can take various different directions. For Nettleton, Neale and Pickering (2013) for example, there is an ambivalence between a desire for normal life and the conviction that normal life is boring. In their analysis of one of their participant's narratives ('and sometimes if I am home and I think this is really boring and shit, I think no, hold on, this is normal life' [ibid: 180]), they argue that the desire for normality is 'the articulation of governmentality with the internalization of the desire not to be marginal' (ibid.). Although this is an interesting analysis from a biopolitical perspective, it does not do justice to the complexity of the desires of the recovering subjectivity, and unwittingly reproduces the 'normative' discourses that it argues against, by associating drug use with a chaotic lifestyle and recovery with stable routines and boredom.

Other empirical studies provide a more complex perspective of the relationship between drug use and normality. Dennis (2019) addresses how one becomes normal *with* drugs, but also how the reality of drug use is not that much about acceleration of speed and a never-ending high, but about the need to perform mundane daily tasks:

> *For Dimitri, drugs are not about becoming-normal, in fact, he explicitly does not wish to be 'normal', but neither are they explicitly about pleasure. Instead, they allowed him to become in a way that made these mundane daily encounters more bearable.*
>
> (Dennis, 2019: 130)

Dennis's analysis resonates with the following account, where the *ability to bear everyday life* and the tasks associated with it, *to bear one-self*, is talked about as an important challenge:

> *I want to be a mature person, independent, stable in my views, with goals, with dreams and to be able to bear, to bear this. To bear to be home alone. To bear to go to work and come back home and to not always think that I'm not good enough, that there's something missing.*

Although in Nettleton, Neale and Pickering's analysis (2013), performing daily, mundane tasks, is considered 'normal' and opposing to the daily life as it is experienced when under the influence of drugs, a close examination of the accounts that address these daily practices do not articulate a desire for normality, but for resistance to a neoliberal way of being, where speed is a requirement.

The accounts of service-users call for a slower pace and argue against the 'normality' of 'having a job', if this is a potential risk for their wellbeing. Being able to bear a stressful life, to resist the acceleration of speed, stay with one-self and take time when making choices, are desires that challenge 'normative' perceptions of worthiness and functionality. The relationship between practices considered 'normal' and the desires of service-users is a complex one, and their segregation is not an easy task, perhaps not even a desirable one. I will now focus on the desire of *becoming slow*, to further emphasise how the recovery assemblage can generate resistance to neoliberal ways of being. In previous chapters, the clash between drug using time and recovery time was addressed as part of the service-users' 'turning up' process. In the accounts that follow, service-users provide a different experience of time, one that is based on slowing down in order to address one-self's needs and make life more bearable.

Becoming slow

Now my aim is to find a job that I like, and I don't want to be exploited. I've got friends that have never done any drugs and their life is all about work, they don't have any personal time ... I don't like that. I don't know, I'd like a job where there are people around, to collaborate in something, something creative maybe. I'm working on it and I think I'll make it, slowly, step by step, I'm not in a hurry.

If I can find some work that I enjoy, I'm not bothered about whether it pays an enormous amount or anything. But what frightens me is being forced into a job that I hate, like I hated working in an office ... that's when I'm at risk again, so I have to try and avoid that somehow. But another one is, if I get like physical exercise outdoors, because I find, I have depression, I like walking around a lot, so you know it would be great if I wanted to be a postman or something! Or do a bit of a work in a park or something, I've done a bit of gardening before. So that's what I want really, is just something where you know I'm reasonably secure in the job and it's not something I hate, then I should be OK. So and then if I've got dreams and aspirations, I can work towards them from a more stable, secure position, but it's just when you've been unemployed for twenty odd years and you're an extreme alcoholic, it's just you've got to take it step by step to get there.

These accounts reflect the concerns of the service-workers discussed earlier, in relation to policymakers' attempts to speed up service-users' 'return to employment'. According to Genie's co-founder, taking time when making choices is essential for one's recovery:

It's OK saying oh anyone can get a job, if we send somebody who's been in active addiction for twenty years and lots of mental health issues and suddenly they're in recovery for three months and then they've got to go and stack shelves in Tesco, they're not going to stay in recovery ... whilst this sounds unfair, if they do some menial jobs, they're less likely to stay in recovery.

There is a negotiation taking place here between two separate priorities: getting a job and maintaining wellbeing. In the first account this conflict is resolved by refusing to unconditionally take any job, and by setting parameters that will simultaneously ensure the service-user's wellbeing ('*I don't want to be exploited*', '*... they don't have any personal time ... I don't like that*', '*I'd like a job where there are people around*'). The way for the accomplishment of this goal is time; doing it slowly, step by step, not being in a hurry. Becoming slow is thus associated with becoming attentive to one's desires, becoming safe, resisting rushed decisions, becoming-well. This perception of time produced in the recovery assemblage clashes with neoliberal time, the fast pace where decisions are made quickly, and people move fast. In other words, the becoming-well clashes with other becomings when extending to other assemblages, and service-users are *at risk again*, as explained in the second account of 'becoming-slow'. Unlike the usual criteria when one looks for a job, it is not money positioned in the focus of attention ('*I'm not bothered about whether it pays an enormous amount or anything*'), but a deeper understanding of one-self and the ability to take their wellbeing into consideration. Doing things slowly, taking it step by step, is presented as essential for the service-user's wellbeing ('*when you've been unemployed for twenty odd years and you're an extreme alcoholic, it's just you've got to take it step by step to get there*'). Therefore, the question of the service-users' agency and ability to make 'healthy' choices is re-introduced under a different prism.

In the previous chapter, the question of individual, 'healthy' choices was complicated and challenged through the provision of examples drawn from service-users' narratives. It was a logic of care, rather than one of choice (Mol, 2008) that better supported their need for the production of new encounters. Practices of care unfolding in the recovery assemblage enabled affective relations that increased the service-users' body's capacity of acting. The accounts of service-users discussed in this chapter express their desire to carry this increased capacity of acting beyond the recovery assemblage. The choices explored – and desired – are the ones that allow the recovery subjectivities to make new meaningful encounters ('*I'd like a job where there are people around, to collaborate in something, something creative maybe*'), even when that entails leaving behind them sets of skills that have been acquired in the past ('*I've trained as a chef but I don't think that I'll choose to continue with that because of the isolation and alienation due to the working hours*'). This reveals a deep sense of self-awareness, not of the individual in isolation, but of the body's capacity of acting, the connections that it needs to make in order to not be at risk, in order to remain 'healthy' ('*When everyone rests I have to work and I don't see how this would be helpful for my recovery if I'm isolated from the people around me*'). Becoming content, becoming slow, becoming connected, express the service-users' desire for their participation in assemblages that render life hopeful, joyful, creative, bearable; assemblages of becoming-well, of always becoming better ('*Just be my best, just be myself and be my best*').

The desire for these assemblages provides strong 'evidence' of the recovering subjectivities' ability to make 'healthy' choices, to care and promote their own wellbeing. What happens though when their wellbeing clashes with the expectations built around the recovery subjectivity? When becoming content does not go hand in hand with becoming employed, when becoming slow is prioritised over becoming fast? The primary question rising from this clash of becomings is 'what constitutes healthy choices?'

We can only start approaching this question once we acknowledge that there are multiple definitions, understandings and ways to talk about 'health'. Following Deleuze and Guattari, I have come to understand 'health' as the resistance of the body to forces of territorialisation (Fox, 2002: 360). In the recovery assemblage, becoming healthy, is made possible through the enablement of affects and relations, 'resisting physical or social territorialisation and experimenting with what is, and what might become. Inevitably, this perspective makes health and health care intrinsically political' (Fox, 2002: 360). The deterritorialisations that started to flow in the recovery assemblage and struggle to extend beyond it are political as they are 'always on the side of freedom, experimentation and becoming, always opposed to power, territory and the fixing of identity' (Fox, 2002: 355). Always thus opposed to neoliberal demands and dominant definitions of health, always pushing the limits of 'what a body can do' and 'what a body can choose'. Following this line of thought, generates a 'politics of health that transcends economic and management perspectives' (Fox, 2002: 361), clashing with current policymaking tendencies in the UK and beyond.

The reterritorialisation and regulation of practices of care, although increasingly more intense and dominating, is not a novel practice but a continuation of the main function of the modern state which is to regulate the decoded, deterritorialised flows and to reterritorialise them, 'so as to prevent the decoded flows from breaking loose at all the edges of the social axiomatic' (Deleuze and Guattari, 1977: 258). Although 'the analysis developed from the work of Deleuze and Guattari suggests an agenda for its practitioners that fosters deterritorialisation in the body-selves of those for whom they care' (Fox, 2002: 361), the two philosophers also stressed that the deterritorialisation of flows of desire is capable of 'demolishing entire social sectors ... It is therefore of vital importance for a society to repress desire, and even to find something more efficient than repression, so that repression, hierarchy, exploitation, and servitude are themselves desired' (Deleuze and Guattari, 1977: 116).

In other words, in the recovery assemblage the body becomes disobedient. Repression, hierarchy, exploitation, and servitude are seen as potentially detrimental for the service-users' wellbeing. Instead, the desire of becoming connected, content and slow tries to extend beyond the recovery assemblage, as a way to maintain and enhance wellbeing. Therefore, the recovering body finds itself in the middle of a conflict; a conflict between the flows of deterritorialised desires, and the forces that struggle to reterritorialise it. Within this conflict, the body of the service-user risks becoming trapped:

Well [after recovery] will be where they keep asking me to prove that I've been looking for work, to show that, I've applied for a certain amount of jobs and then with that comes the pressure, well if you're not making enough of an effort we're going to have to sanction you and all this sort of stuff. So I'm not looking forward to that ... I've kind of proved that I'm fit for work now because I've got certificates and stuff, I've done courses you know that show that I'm employable now, and I've you know updated my CV ... So I'm proving me self-confident all the time, so the more I do that, the less likely I'll be able to get away with, if you like claiming sick ... You can't just run before you can walk, you've got to go as far as you can at your own pace and if the authorities are willing to let you get away with it! So I've been quite lucky so far but you know I'm getting to the end of, I can't just keep pre-empting them anymore, I can't just keep doing courses, I can't get away with it anymore, I know that it's going to get to a point now where I've got to do this, this and this and there's no way round it and, so there's some trepidation but it's better than going back to the way I was before, and I don't think, you just can't rely on the Benefits system anymore, it's a complete shambles at the moment ... Because really, let's face it, to be dependent on Benefits now, you'd need a time machine (laughs) I mean I laugh but it's not funny like you know.

This is just a small insight into a service-user's relationship with the benefit's system. His willing participation in the courses provided for the development of skills has ensured that he could get the support he needed (payment of his allowance would have been stopped if he had refused to take the courses). Additionally, some were courses that did enhance his skills and grasped his interest, as he would quite often report when coming into Genie. At the same time, they entrapped him as he has now '*proved that [he's] fit for work because [he's] got certificates and stuff*'. Does this image of a self-confident, employable person describe his everyday reality? As a chronic alcoholic and having suffered with depression for years, having a job that he has not taken the time to choose based on his needs and desires, could be detrimental for his physical and mental health. And the complexities in the story of the specific service-user go deeper. Finally, his engagement with Genie is a proof that he is addressing his alcohol consumption – which he has indeed minimised during his time at Genie – rendering him even more 'employable'. Overall, it is his desire to make new connections that 'proves' he is 'fit for work'. The paradox being addressed here is that the desire of becoming-well, when extending beyond the recovery assemblage, re-positions the wellbeing of the service-users at risk. While the affective flows produced in the recovery assemblage pave the way for an understanding of 'work' as a field where novel connections could be made possible, the pressure to 'get a job' and 'get on with it' reterritorialises these lines of flight and creates a vicious circle where service-users are confronted with the same issues that blocked their flows of desire at first place:

> *It's really hard to find a job and there's lots of exploitation and that creates problems. Guys [service-users] finish the programme and they say fine, I'm recovered alright, is this how my life is going to be? So essentially they confront again the same problems, the same reasons they started using at first place.*

> *Employers these days don't look for employees, they look for multi-machines. A driver who's IT literate and speaks three languages and if they also have first aid training even better! As you can imagine people that have been in addiction have missed out on educational opportunities ... Unemployment in Greece is very high and most businesses don't hire people, especially not people that they'd have to train.*

The statements above of two therapists of 18 ano highlight that even though the social and financial circumstances differ, service-users in both Athens and Liverpool are at risk of having their desires reterritorialised, once extended beyond the recovery assemblage. For UK-based service-users, policymaking time clashes with recovery time by pushing people towards employment without taking into consideration how this might be detrimental for their wellbeing. Accordingly, in Greece, service-users are expected to re-integrate in a labour market defined by relationships of exploitation deriving from a long-term financial crisis. In both cases, the desire of becoming-slow is being reterritorialised by a system that emerges in everyday practices of speed and intensity. 'Liberated' from their relationship with substances, the bodies considered 'recovered' are expected to become part of this system, even if, more than the substance, it is the speed of the world that makes them ill.

This takes us back to an earlier discussion, where service-users addressed the need for an 'extension' of the recovery assemblage. Some of them talked about recovery as a 'way of being' (and doing), others suggested a prolonged recovery process that would ensure their smooth transition back to the social, and in some cases, it was imagined how work could become a milieu for the deterritorialisation of the affective flows produced in the recovery assemblage. Underlying all these narratives there is an urgent call for the redefinition of recovery. As already mentioned, the need for an extension of the recovery assemblage should in no way be perceived as an embodiment of medicalisation or other approaches that depart from the conviction 'once an addict always an addict'. More than anything, the desire for the extension of the recovery assemblage beyond the space and time of recovery reveals a desire for long-standing and sustainable wellbeing. It is an internalised through lived experiences conviction that a body does not just become well but is always *becoming well*; there are no 'recovered' but *recovering bodies*; bodies that are not interested in being 'cured' in isolation in order to be 'functional', but desire a wellbeing that is always becoming through the connections with other assemblages that keep enhancing a body's capacity to act. It is when these connections are broken that bodies become at risk of collapsing, and the question of 'relapse' emerges.

Relapse: connections built and broken

'Relapse prevention' is a familiar concept and practice for those engaged with drug treatment services. The ways that 'relapse prevention' is currently practised and talked about draws primarily on research produced within the discipline of psychology, and especially by researchers and practitioners adopting cognitive behavioural (Marlatt and Donovan, 2005; Witkiewitz and Marlatt, 2009) and neurocognitive approaches (Tapert et al., 2004). The outcome has been the production of 'tools' and 'mechanisms', put in place to 'prevent' people from relapsing. This has generated the assumption that once access to these 'tools' has been granted, relapse becomes a problem of the individual, a personal 'success' or 'failure', a measurement of how much one 'really' wants to recover. This system of thought reproduces long standing discourses of blame against drug users and fuels the discussion on the 'revolving doors' of recovery (White and Kelly, 2010), holding treatment services accountable for 'failing' to produce and maintain 'recovered' bodies.

In the chapter 'Becoming a drug user – becoming a service-user', the Deleuzian 'turning point' was mobilised to account for the desire of becoming-other, flowing through substances. I then discussed how encounters with care gradually lead towards another 'turning point', the engagement with services, when substances come to block the desires of becoming. I will now account for a third 'turning point', that of relapse, the moment that the service-user returns to the substance for a shorter or longer period of time. My aim is to challenge the production of relapse as an individual problem and failure of service-users and treatment services, and to rethink it as *a desire to connect*, a desire that can be either enhanced, or broken. Relapse is investigated in two different ways. Initially I approach it as part of the temporality of recovery, a way to start building connections with services; as the expression of an emerging desire under exploration. Drawing on Deleuze's philosophy of temporality (1994), recovery is conceived not 'as a distinct process in and of itself but rather a series of processes that come to generate different modalities of time' (Bristow, 2018: 75). Bringing together the narratives of people in recovery with Deleuze's (1994) syntheses of time, 'relapse time' is addressed as an intrinsic part of the recovery assemblage, a constitutive element of the modifications, differences and repetitions (Deleuze, 1994) that render new connections desirable and possible. Secondly, I will discuss relapse as the consequence of broken and interrupted connections when policy fails to support the encounters emerging in the recovery space, disrupting thus the recovery process. Drawing on Garcia's (2010) analysis of the entanglement between historico-political spaces and chronicity, relapse is discussed as the outcome of the interrupted relationship between a subject and a recovery space.

Although addressing the reasons behind the service-users' relapses is of high importance for the improvement of the practices of care provided by services, the intention here is to discuss relapse not as a failure, but as part of the *recovering assemblage*. Up until now I have mobilised the term *recovery assemblage*, to address the specific material, affective and social assemblages of Genie and 18 ano. Following the previous argument on an understanding of recovery as a state of always becoming, I introduce the term *recovering assemblage* in order to verbalise this perception of the recovery body as becoming. While the *recovery assemblage* has specific territorial and occasionally temporal components, the *recovering assemblage* entails all the encounters that a body produces before, during and after its engagement with a specific recovery assemblage. These include all the affective encounters (harm reduction practices, relationships of care while using, turning points) that precede one's engagement with recovery services, as well as all the encounters that proceed it (becoming content, connected, slow and reterritorialised). This way of thinking draws theoretically on McLeod's (2017) analysis of wellbeing as a non-linear, complex process that takes illbeing and destratification seriously, and empirically on the service-users' narratives, whose experiences of recovery transcend the territorial component of the recovery assemblage. Thinking with the recovering assemblage we might be able to better understand and support service-users from their first experiences of drug use, to their destratification and engagement with one or various services, to their relapses and reterritorialisation, and hopefully enable the deterritorialisation of their becomings made possible in the recovery assemblage.

Relapse and the desire for connection

In *Difference and Repetition*, Deleuze (1994) produces an ontology of time and memory through three interrelated and interactive syntheses of time. The first one is the passive synthesis of the living present, where 'through contraction, past events and future possibilities become actualised in the present moment' (Bristow, 2018: 75). The past, present and future are conceptualised through *repetition*, the experience of expectancy produced by things that happened 'before', leading to expectations about the processes of the future (ibid.). The second synthesis, the passive synthesis of the pure past, accords to *memory* and how it informs present temporal processes, while the last one, the static synthesis of the future, is able to create a *difference*, 'to impact upon the present and the past by remaining open' (ibid: 76–77). By following accounts of people in recovery with Deleuze's conceptualisation of time, I explore how the connections built in the recovery space allow for an understanding of the repetition of relapse and its memory, as a process that renders *different becomings* possible, 'offering practical insights into the [recovering] subject's emergence' (Duff and Price-Robertson, 2018: 98).

> *I've come to realise that all the years that I've been using, I've also been trying to quit.*

'Turning points' have been discussed as ruptures with time, as well as processes that lead to a desire for new becomings. The statement of the service-user above articulates this complexity; this conflict between contradictory desires challenges the simplification of subjectivities by imagining a direct link between a body's desires and actions. Conversely, it is indicative of the conflicts, contradictions and complexities that traverse a body's flows of desire. It also paves the way for the understanding of the recovering body not only as the one engaging with a specific service, but as a body that carries the desire of recovering, whether this is acted upon or not.

Acknowledging the complexity of the recovering assemblage and the conflicting desires that it entails is fundamental if we are committed to shifting away from discourses of blame (against the services and the users) to the understanding of the recovering body as a modification (Deleuze, 1994: 70), affective and affected by the assemblages that it encounters. Deleuze's work on Hume's thesis that '*[r]epetition changes nothing in the object repeated, but does change something in the mind which contemplates it*' (1994: 70) is useful here for the analysis of service-users' experiences of re-presenting at the same service:

> *I didn't take their help straight away. Nor did I trust them straightaway. It was very hard for me, hence I came for a second time. I had lots of issues. One time was not enough.*

> *When I called the first time I hadn't understood what they do. It was like, since I couldn't escape from the whole thing [referring to personal problems] through using [drugs] then I'd go there [to the programme]. And that's why I didn't stay. I freaked out. I was 22 … This had to do with me, the situation I was in. I didn't go to quit [drugs]. [I wanted to] find another way to leave from what was going on at home, because the way I'd found [drug use] was killing me.*

These are reflections of the body as a modification, accounts of people's first experiences of the recovery encounter, narrated while they are re-engaging with the same service. The affective relations produced through a body's encounter with a recovery service differ, following its becomings. So, while the service remains the same, repetition changes 'something in the mind that contemplates it' (Deleuze, 1994: 70), enabling the becoming of affective relations that were not made possible through the first encounter. Reading re-presentation as a failure of the users does not address the complexity of their desire of becoming-other. Accordingly, blaming a service for not instantly producing 'recovered' bodies does not enable a closer look at the small gestures, the minor modifications that eventually rendered the second encounter – and potentially long-lasting one – possible. It should thus be acknowledged that *all encounters between the service and the user matter*, and constitute components of an ongoing turning point that gradually enables connections between the using body and the recovering assemblage, opening up the way for a future deterritorialisation.

These connections are not always visible or straightforward and in many cases service-users emphasised that they could not have talked 'back then' the way they talk 'now'. The narratives of the service-users take place at a present time where the past and the future are dimensions of this present (Deleuze, 1994: 76).

> *A scar is the sign not of a past wound but of 'the present fact of having been wounded': we can say that it is the contemplation of the wound, that it contracts all the instants which separate us from it into a living present.*
>
> (Deleuze, 1994: 77)

In the descriptions shared in this book, service-users contemplate the fact of having been wounded and imagine a future, while becoming with the recovery assemblage. They are not subjects emerging 'before time, or even contemporaneous with it, rather the subject is in and of time; a form of unfolding time and its divergent syntheses' (Duff and Price-Robertson, 2018: 102).

Therefore, the primary aim of recovery is not the provision of 'relapse prevention' and 'coping' tools, but the enhancement of the connections that render the contemplation of wounds possible, and the desire of becoming-other stronger. By positioning the focus on the connections that become possible within the recovery space, healing becomes a sociopolitical rather than an individual process, 'accomplished less through personal therapeutics and processing of painful memories than through a small-scale, tentative restoration of ties of trust and support' (Biehl and Locke, 2010: 334). It is in the recovering assemblage that a body's capacity to act is both enhanced and protected, creating space and time for the contemplation of the past and an imagination of the future. It is this present becoming that renders possible the contemplation of past encounters and how these matter, either with the same service, as discussed earlier, or with different services, as talked about in what follows:

But the thing with it was, it did help me, because it did actually put me on the rung to like, you know the right path if you like, but there wasn't enough going on for me, I still had far too much time, which you know for me was an absolute killer, the isolation, I needed to be involved. And I put this to him [keyworker] one day, and he suggested a few other organisations.

That was better, there was a lady there that, she was, she understood some of it, she'd had you know similar experiences, and she was actually from Norway, which is where my eldest daughter's from, and we engaged because we had contacts with, through Norway and that was something where you know her life and mine actually touched. So yeah, that was a little more personal and I was more interested in that, but I eventually slipped back into drink. After two, two and a half months or so.

I'd tried many times [to engage with recovery] but I wasn't ready, I didn't want to get into this when I was younger. Maybe in the back of my head I did but with every failed attempt I'd see I'm not ready ... at the age of 35 I realised that I had to do something, that I was in danger and I would either live or die.

Service-users reflect on the encounters that slowly enabled their 'present' connection with a service; they reflect on their experience of the recovering assemblage. These encounters take all kinds of different shapes and forms. They might have put someone on '*the right path*', where '*right*' here stands for the support provided to the service-user to identify his needs and move on to another service ('*I needed to be involved. And I put this to him [keyworker] one day, and he suggested a few other organisations*'). For another service-user it was his encounter and connection with another person that enabled his first recovery experience ('*there was a lady there that, she was, she understood some of it, she'd had you know similar experiences*'), while in the third account, the service-user talks about the desire of recovery being somewhere at the back of her head, leading to failed attempts until she felt ready to establish a long-standing connection with a service. Overall, service-users share their experiences of 'testing the waters' of recovery, until the desire of becoming a service-user prevails over the desire of becoming a user. In their narratives the emphasis is on *time*, and encounters that get blocked or render other connections possible. Thinking of re-presentation and engagement with various services as articulations of different encounters within the recovering assemblage, challenges discourses of blame. The body that re-presents at a service is always becoming, never the same as the one that approached the service the first time. It is between these repetitions that difference lies (Deleuze, 1994: 76) and recovery becomes possible.

Engaging with different services and experimenting with various ways of connecting until the encounter that unblocks a body's flow of desire is mobilised, is an essential component of the recovering assemblage. This was stressed by all workers in Genie and 18 ano. Although both services are recovery-focused, and thus their members of staff would be 'categorised' as advocates of recovery and abstinence, they all emphasised that all possible treatment approaches should be available to service-users, from harm reduction services to different types of recovery. Accordingly, those categorised as harm reduction 'advocates' share the same views, as discussed with one of the members of the team that operated the first harm reduction service in Liverpool:

> a lot of it is about making the person happier and safer as an individual so they can actually cope with either staying on methadone long term or coming of it eventually for reduction. So I think all harm reductionists believe that a range of options to come off should be available ... it's highly complex and everybody is different so I think really it's flexibility and the ability of approaches that's important giving to people if you can afford it, a lot of different options for staying on methadone or harm reduction approach or coming off in different ways.

The belief that all types of services and approaches should be available, expressed by all workers that I encountered and who follow the (recovering) users' everyday realities, repositions the question of time and agency in the focus of attention: there is using time, harm reduction time, recovery time, and accordingly relapse time, all of them part of the recovering assemblage. It is the service-users, through their encounters in the assemblages within which they operate, that can better decide how their desire of becoming-other can be addressed, when and if they will transition from one time to another. This emphasises the necessity of existence of practices of care throughout all these different timings, and directly challenges the need for 'central drug policies' that attempt to control the using and recovering time, by prioritising certain treatment approaches over others. Focusing on practices of care collaboratively created, rather than the regulation of the way harm reduction and recovery is done, renders possible the enablement of potential turning points throughout one's encounter with a substance, encouraging a meaningful engagement with services that do not attempt to control using and recovering bodies, but to enhance their capacity to act.

Relapse and broken connections

Relapse and re-presentation to services has been addressed as a component of the recovering assemblage, when through the narratives of the service-users it is discussed as part of a body's modification through its shifting encounters with one or various services. Following Deleuze's (1994) conceptualisation of temporality, 'relapse time' becomes one of the temporalities of the recovering process. However, for relapse to be addressed in all its complexity, accounting for the connections produced is not enough; we also need to account for the connections broken. I do so by shifting my attention from time to space, drawing on Garcia's (2010) analysis of the entanglement between historico-political spaces and chronicity.

In her ethnography *The Pastoral Clinic: Addiction and Dispossession along the Rio Grande*, Garcia (2010) explores how New Mexico's landscape and addiction are shaped together, narrating a shared story of mourning and loss. Through this entanglement, 'institutional structures and claims are absorbed by the addict, exacerbating a sense of personal failure that contributes to a collective sense of hopelessness and, in turn, the regional heroin problem itself' (Garcia, 2010: 8–9), unfolding the problem of 'chronicity' not as a medical one, but as a sociopolitical issue. Addressing Deleuze's question on the causality of drug use (2007) and whether its transformation from a vital experimentation into deadly dependence is inevitable, Garcia focuses on the context within which repetition is produced: the historico-political space of Rio Grande where the outcome of repetition always remains the same, and difference is always blocked from becoming. Garcia's subject is not unitary; it emerges in the flux of time, affects and relations (Duff and Price-Robertson, 2018: 98). While though in the accounts discussed earlier this emergence was becoming through modifications and novel connections that open up new possibilities for difference, in Rio Grande the (addicted) subject is trapped in repetition and broken connections, constituted by feelings of loss and mourning (Vitellone, 2015: 383–384).

Rio Grande's historico-political space drives Garcia's analysis of the detoxification space where her participants' attempts to 'go clean' are trapped in repetition. Drawing on Garcia's emphasis on space, I return to relapse and the empirical accounts of service-users to discuss how the symbolic space of policy affects the connections built in the material space of recovery. In the empirical accounts that follow, it is policy that blocks the possibility of difference, by breaking the connections produced in the recovering assemblage. I explore how relapse is talked about as an outcome of policy and systemic failures, deriving from the domination of a medical apparatus opting for short-lived and fragmentary interventions. Unlike the narratives discussed earlier, where the desire for connections was emerging, the following accounts show how the recovering subjectivity is affected when the connections enabled through the recovering assemblage break, the body's becoming-other is interrupted, and the desire of becoming a user re-emerges:

> *I was only really being seen for a couple of weeks or something and then the support went. And then there was a couple of times I had breakdowns and the first time they ran tests in the hospital and stuff but again, I was discharged after a short while, I didn't you know stay in hospital at all. And then I went to the doctors with, again anxiety, depression kind of issues,*

and I did the cognitive behavioural therapy, the talking therapy, but again that only lasted a couple of weeks. So there was nothing really long-term, structured or disciplined or anything like that until I got referred to Genie.

I started engaging with services probably about twenty years ago and I was engaged with one and I didn't find it useful or the funding stopped or they closed down.

At first, when I first started drinking, I was around twenty one, and that went on till like I was about twenty two, so it was about a year, and then I tried this rehab place … and I ended up doing that for eight months, a residential rehab. And then once I completed that, I came back to Liverpool and I, you know stayed like sober for a couple of months but because I'd made all like my connections there, I come back to Liverpool and then you know, I had no like friends or connections, so I picked up again and went out there for like another eight years on and off.

The first account discusses the engagement with different institutions for short periods of time, until '*the support went*'. The narrative follows medical encounters at the hospital and with one's GP and psychological encounters through CBT and talking therapy. All these encounters were interrupted ('*nothing really long-term, structured or disciplined*'), breaking the connections that would have potentially led to a different investment of the service-user's desire. This narrative resonates with Gomart's criticism of specialists' apparatuses that, instead of acknowledging that the problem lies with them for failing to acknowledge relapse as a phenomenon in which they are supposed to intervene, they instead attribute relapse to the patient's difficulty to commit to a human relation with the therapist (2004: 91). The difficulty then discussed through this narrative is produced by the way that the medical space is produced. Following short medical and psychological interventions the 'patient' is discharged, considered recovered, and the connection with a potentially recovering space is interrupted, blocking possibilities of difference.

Accordingly, in the second account, both types of 'relapse' are addressed. Occasionally services were not found useful, but in other cases, '*the funding stopped or they closed down*'. Once more, the connections made possible appear to be unexpectedly interrupted, leaving the desire of becoming-other un-addressed. The third account discusses the lack of aftercare in the community, following the completion of a residential rehabilitation programme. Although the service-user managed to successfully attend and complete the programme, the connections created were interrupted when that ended, leaving him in isolation.

This interruption of connections is addressed by both service-users and workers, and traverses different types of support services. In a conversation with a social worker that used to work at 18 ano and now manages a residential service for young people in London, the process of making connections that are interrupted due to the fact that residents are expected to 'move on' when they turn 18, was talked about as potentially responsible for young people's isolation in the community:

There are kids that stay with us [at the service] and have significant mental health or addiction issues, or comorbidity and if they could stay with us until the age of 20, with the relationship that we'd have developed with them and with the work being done, because an adolescent does not connect easily, at the age of 19-20 [they] might be able to connect with therapy, but when at the age of 18 this provision is cut and they tell them go live in a flat on your own and make your own connections with the services and the community because we have to save money, there you see that it is the financial management that defines the case management.

The experience of this social worker demonstrates that although the desire for the development of encounters that can enhance a body's capacity to act is present from both workers and service-users, it is eventually blocked by the space of policy, through decisions that derive from financial imperatives, not taking into consideration the lived experiences of those that work at, and those that benefit from the specific service. The examples of cases where the financial management, together with policymaking decisions that do not develop organically lead to the reterritorialisation of the connections built vary, and affect the care provided in diverse ways. This is demonstrated by the account below, where the co-founder of Genie discussed how, when the service was still funded by the Council, it had to comply with a never-ending shift of the goalposts:

So for instance, Liverpool City Council might say to us one year, we want you to engage 75% of people with alcohol issues and 25% with drug issues, and the next year they change the goalposts ... You know so suddenly we needed to engage 60% of clients on methadone rather than 75% with alcohol. So the profile of clients changed when the funders changed their criteria ... [But] where there's a will there's a way! And most people cross-addict, there's not many people who, who are just heroin users and have never had a problem with alcohol or they've stopped the heroin, the alcohol becomes an issue ... So somebody will present to you as a heroin user and you say, well do you have an issue with alcohol, no. If you dig a little bit deeper they'll go, yeah, actually I do, and it's the minute I don't have my gear on me I'll drink three bottles of wine, so statistics, schmistics! [laughs] But that said, it still had a detrimental effect I think on the development of Genie, because whilst you can be quite cute with it as well, in that respect, which everybody does, we still did need to have that focus on something else. So for instance, when we had to engage 75% heroin and methadone users, we set up so much outreach at Merseycare, we used to go to Merseycare once a month, we'd be in their reception, where most people presenting to them have got enduring heroin use. So we built all these links up and then, ooh, we don't want you to do that now, we want you to do alcohol. So suddenly all that work you've done for those twelve months and built all these relationships up has gone, because then you're moving over to the alcohol nurse in the hospital. So it's detrimental I think to move the goalposts. I do think there's ways around it, but you can't just ignore what your funders are asking you for. So whilst you're working on implementing those ways around it, you're not supporting your clients as much.

The above is an in-depth account of the balance between abiding by a funder's criteria and prioritising the needs of service-users. Whilst, '*where there is a will there is a way*', damage is done when the connections built between the service and the community are broken, the effect can be detrimental. Constantly looking for '*ways around*' the shifting goalposts takes time and energy, eventually affecting the support provided to service-users. The recovering spaces built through connections with other services and the communities are dismantled when policy intervenes and the goalposts change. While the service changes its practices in order to address the new goalposts, the emergence of subjectivities produced in repetition and difference is interrupted.

Troubling relapse

What good does it do to perceive as fast as a quick-flying bird if speed and movement continue to escape somewhere else?

(Deleuze and Guattari, 2004: 314)

Lapses, parapraxes and symptoms are like birds that strike their beaks against the window. It is not a question of interpreting them. It is a question instead of identifying their trajectory to see if they can serve as indicators of new universes or reference capable of acquiring a consistency sufficient for turning a situation upside down.

(Guattari quoted in Deleuze, 1998: 63–64)

For Deleuze and Guattari, drug users are like quick-flying birds, producing assemblages whose speed and movement escape somewhere else, failing to deterritorialise the flows of desire that traverse them. Conversely, lapses, parapraxes and symptoms are not about speed and movement, but about persistence; birds striking their beaks against the window, demanding visibility. This metaphor challenges the production of relapse as an 'indicator of a pathological determination by a memorializing unconscious' (Biehl and Locke, 2010: 332). Following Deleuze and Guattari, relapse has been addressed through the narratives of people in recovery and service-workers, as an indicator of new universes capable of turning a situation upside down. Drawing on the words of Guattari, relapse is unfolded as an urgency for connections, a potentiality of new becomings (Biehl and Locke, 2010: 332). I have followed this desire for connections and new becomings as they are enhanced and blocked inside and beyond the recovering assemblage. Initially I focused on how service-users discuss their first engagement with services, talking about this encounter as an exploration of the connections that could be made possible. This process is not linear, and relapse is very often part of it. Thinking of relapse as entangled with the recovering process, part of its temporality and an act of repetition that renders difference possible, challenges its pathologisation. Conversely, it is a testimony of the fact that all recovering encounters matter, as they carry a desire for wellbeing, where wellbeing does not stand for a stable state, a final goal to be achieved, but a non-linear, complex process of becoming, entangled with illbeing and destratifications (McLeod, 2017). Challenging narratives of recovery where the 'recovered' subject emerges as stable and fixed, it is small gestures, occasionally interrupted by relapses and renegotiations with one's desire of becoming a service-user that establish long-term meaningful connections that enhance a body's capacity to act.

Relapse has also been explored as the outcome of policy's failure to enable the longevity of the connections made possible in the recovering assemblage. When financial management is prioritised over case management, connections are broken and service-users are left in isolation, dislocated from the spaces of recovery where difference is becoming. The striking beaks against the window are ignored and people in recovery are trapped in repetitions with similar outcomes. The space of policy is thus exposed as *disconnected* from the recovering realities of the subjects it is called to care for. The need that arises is the reconnection of policy practices with the lived experiences of recovery, the practice of policy as a force focused on strengthening rather than blocking the connections built within the recovering space, a force that increases the possibilities of difference, emerging through repetition. Thinking with relapse demonstrates the need to closely explore how the interruption of connections affects the realities of people in recovery. This need is reflected in the present analysis of the recovering assemblage, and has also been observed and criticised by empirical studies on harm reduction that have focused on how bad connections or the lack of them cost lives (Dennis, 2019: 135).

Relapse has been unpacked as one of the components that contribute to the wider question of how we can do recovery differently; how we can understand recovery as a desire for connections, and what is the role of policy in enhancing and enabling this flow of desire. Thinking with the Deleuzo–Guattarian assemblage unfolds the practice of recovery as a series of processes caring not for the production of 'recovered' individuals, but for the enablement of new becomings and desires. Finally, my attempt has been to explore how relapse is made in practice and in policy, and most importantly how it can be made differently, how can we enable the striking beaks against the window to be better heard and attended?

In this last chapter, I have addressed the reterritorialisations that service-users are called to fight against in their attempts to extend the flows of the desires becoming in the recovery assemblage, to other social assemblages. Dominant policymaking practices, emerging outside the recovery assemblage, have been discussed as reterritorialising forces that fail to address the service-users' desire for the enhancement of life possibilities. In the conclusion, it is further explored how the interruption of connections affects the care provided by services, and the deterritorialisations becoming within the spaces of recovery. Finally, I imagine how policy could be done otherwise, more carefully, entangled with the practices emerging *inside* the recovery assemblage.

Conclusion

Services interrupted

In August 2019 Genie had to close its doors. Following the cut of its governmental funding in 2016, and after three years of constant bids to different funders, all sources of money had been exhausted. Despite the efforts of the founder and the manager to explore alternative funding options, the service had to eventually close.

Members of staff were made aware of the upcoming closure of the service a few days before it was announced to the service-users. They were asked to not share any information with them, until the right support was in place to help service-users go through this period of uncertainty. Genie's workers had to be as present and supportive as always, while dealing with the emotional and the practical implications of the service's closure. I experienced the consequences of this precarious state before, when in 2012 I was training in art therapy at 18 ano, at a time when the future not only of one recovery service, but of the whole public health system in Greece was up in the air. While the engagement of 18 ano with the anti-austerity movement enabled the production of vital connections inside and outside the recovery assemblage, the uncertainty regarding the future of the service, affected the everyday realities of the workers:

> *The memory of the degradation of public health and of course mental health is still very fresh and that had a direct impact on the clinical work ... It was like we are all a vulnerable population, service-users and service workers trying to compose a common stance towards it [threat of closure].*

The loss of jobs for service workers and the impact on their daily lives when their working conditions are deteriorated is a major issue which does not only affect them as individuals, but impacts on the connections enabled in the recovery assemblage; but the focus here is on how the degradation or closure of services reterritorialises the service-users' desires. The following are examples of reterritorialisation, when the connections nurtured in the recovery assemblage are broken or interrupted.

DOI: 10.4324/9781003165613-9

Most drug and alcohol services in the UK are obliged to only accept service-users coming from certain postcodes. For example, if a person lives in a L1 postcode area of Liverpool they cannot engage with services with L8 postcodes. Apart from the obvious problems and exclusions that this system creates, especially for homeless people and those without stable accommodation, it also significantly diminishes the treatment options available, as the users are not free to choose a service based on its approach, but on its location, applying in practice Deleuze and Guattari's (1977) view that policy 'codes' the flows of desire. Genie used to take pride in being able to accept everyone, no matter what their postcode was, as talked about by one of the keyworkers:

> on the fact of simple things like that, postcodes lots of little things that irritate, that aggravate, and create anxiety for these guys … I got it when I was a client and I got it when I was working in it. Postcodes don't affect here. There's no barrier to come to Genie, you can come from anywhere, and these guys, it's Liverpool-only, Sefton-only these borders that don't really exist. They're all barriers to recovery. Services talk a lot about building bridges. I spent two and a half years trying to do that and still struggle with some of them.

With Genie's closure, the barrier of postcodes re-presented. After a meeting with all members of staff and service-users, where the upcoming closure of Genie was announced, I facilitated with the keyworker a recovery group, aimed at initiating a discussion on the options that were available to the service-users. During this group, it was not the desired connections – or how people felt about them being interrupted – that drove the conversation, but postcodes. Most of the participants were aware of the services available within their postcode area. Some people had already engaged with them at different occasions, and quite a few felt that these services had not been able to meet their needs. The discussion subsequently focused on services that are 'flexible' when it comes to postcodes, and specific workers that would potentially be willing to turn a blind eye and accept service-users from different areas. This was considered by everyone in the group a very important, urgent issue, and it is within the recovery groups that practical problems like this have to be addressed and resolved. However, this example comes to demonstrate how within an hour, the enhancement of affective relations within a service was interrupted, and a practical obstacle came to dominate the group.

The process that led to Genie's closure was long and started in 2016 when the service lost its public funding. As the founder of Genie explains this was not a 'personal' decision against the service, or based on the 'results' or 'evidence of success' provided, but a side effect of reduction of funding that led to the council allocating all the available resources to one big service rather than multiple smaller ones:

well the reason is that there was a massive reduction in money from central government to local government, so it wasn't a personal reason to Genie ... So thirty-nine people [services], us being one of them, lost their contracts. And that was purely based on less money that local government had and to streamline it, they just wanted one large national statutory provider, which means they're only dealing with one organisation ... We did have a choice, it wasn't like, we're taking your funding off you, that's it, we were one of three [services] where they said, we're taking your funding off you, we're giving it to this large national organisation but you can go and work for them if you want to ... So we had many meetings with the large national organisation for them to sub-contract us but still keep the premises, still keep the name and still keep the delivery and the culture of Genie, but that just wasn't an option ... So it felt to us that it would not be what we deliver, you know, it's not what we're passionate about, there's no informed choices, it's a clinical organisation, people go there because they're court ordered to a lot of the time, so it doesn't have the welcoming atmosphere Genie has, simply because it's attached to probation and the prison. So it's needed, I'm not saying it's not needed, but it's not the only thing that's needed.

While a lot of work has been done towards the criticism of policy documents and recommendations (McKeganey, 2007; Reuter and Stevens, 2007; Room, 2004), the challenges that services deal with in their daily operations extend beyond this way of understanding policymaking. The narration of Genie's founder requires that we take a few steps back, and instead of focusing on the provision of another set of policy recommendations, we question what 'policy' entails. It requires the acknowledgment of the gap between the design of policy in theory and its implementation in practice, and a conscious shift from the understanding of policy as a governmental task to *policy as practice* emerging from the relations produced within the recovery assemblage, and the deterritorialisations made possible through these encounters:

when the drug treatment strategy came out in 2010, I was quite new to this field, so four years into it, and I read the drug treatment strategy and I was elated, I thought, brilliant, Genie's going to get so much funding, because it was like it had been written for us. It was recovery focused, it was about informed choices, it was about wellbeing ... I thought well we're fine, we're going to get loads of money, no problem. But to trickle down from the top government in London to the commissioners in Liverpool, they've lost it by the time it gets to them ... So when it comes to changing policy, yeah, it would be great to see policy change, what would be even better would be to see it implemented. They're changing it all the time.

In the account above, as well as through quotes discussed in the previous chapter, service workers share their experiences of constant changes in policy, either through shifting the focus of attention on different using populations (alcohol users, heroin users etc.) or through prioritising harm reduction over recovery and vice versa. These changes are occasionally detrimental for the connections that each specific recovery assemblage has already built, or in other cases, the workers find ways around them. However, what does not seem to change, is the reterritorialisation of the flows of desire produced in each service, through politics that attempt to 'code' and moderate the practices of care developed organically. One of the main commitments of this book has been to render visible the deterritorialisations becoming possible in the recovery assemblage, and subsequently expose how these are blocked.

The emergence of policies as fully formed, coherent and stable 'things' has already been convincingly contested (McCann and Ward, 2012). According to McCann and Ward, policies 'are assemblages of parts of the near and far, of fixed and mobile pieces of expertise, regulation, institutional capacities, etc. that are brought together in particular ways and for particular interests and purposes' (2012: 328). What this book's analysis has brought to the thinking of the policy assemblage is policy's entanglement with care. Following the lived experiences of service-users and workers, I have attended to the *becoming of policy within the recovery assemblage*, and as a practice of care. This way of thinking and doing policy is an ethical and political imperative extending beyond spaces of recovery, and challenging neoliberal systems of thought and time. By paying attention to the service-users' voices the aim has not been to question or praise the process of recovery, but to closely attend to the connections that we build or break in all the assemblages within which we operate.

Following the service-users' desire of becoming-other, the aim is to make visible how the collaborating services *care for these shifting desires*, how they enhance their flow. Care and desire have been theoretically, methodologically and empirically entangled. Drawing on feminist analyses and problematisations of care, following people's shifting desires has been put forward as a caring research practice. This approach called for attention to the service-users' *desire for care*, as this was unfolded through their narratives, as well as to the services' *desire to care* for their service-users, as this was unpacked through the close examination of the practices of care in place. In so doing, policy, and how it is understood and experienced by service-users and workers has been revealed as a force that blocks the flows of desire enhanced in the recovery assemblage.

Although the empirical accounts of this interruption of flows of desire refer to the recent past and present of services, they also reflect how policy interventions have been historically experienced by drug and alcohol services. In the chapter 'Of other spaces: the birth of the heterotopia of recovery', the history of Genie was discussed in parallel with the history of harm reduction and other recovery UK services. What holds these histories together is their inclusion and exclusion from the allocation of public funding, depending on their ability and willingness to adjust their approaches and practices according to governmentally designed policy strategies and goals. The way policy is discussed in this book attempts to go beyond specific drug and alcohol treatment strategies and approaches. What is being problematised is the 'logic of policy' overall.

Deleuze and Guattari have given us the tools to unpack the difficult connection between recovery as a policy and as a practice. Understanding recovery as an assemblage, opens up a new way of thinking about policy. This is not a statement against policy overall, but against policy being formulated *outside* the recovery assemblage, disconnected from the desires of service-users. As explained by the manager of Genie, the problem starts when policy decisions are made elsewhere and do not emerge from, or attempt to develop any connections with the recovery assemblage:

> *I think the government is not looking at what's happening on the ground. I think in funding they look at dotting I's and crossing T's, what looks good on paper, but they're not out there and seeing how it affects people on a day to day basis. I think they're out of touch on how they fund.*

The necessity that derives is a shift of attention from the *outside* to the *inside* of the assemblage, and more specifically to policy, as it happens and grows organically through the encounters and affective practices unfolded in the everyday reality of the recovery practice. In other words, caring practices *are* policy in action, yet neglected in how funding is allocated.

Paying attention to the 'inside' of the drug treatment assemblage, more often than not leads to the rejection of the oppositional dynamic between recovery and harm reduction treatment models (Dennis, Rhodes and Harris, 2020), and to a focus instead on how recovery (or harm reduction) is daily negotiated and practised. Dennis and colleagues' (2020) exploration of 'movement' in UK drug services, exposes both narrow and absolute, as well as open and flexible recovery practices, emerging in the same service. These analyses further accentuate the urgency of a close exploration of recovery practices in place, and how these can inform policymaking approaches that derive from existing caring practices.

The previous chapter primarily focused on how service-users attempt to find ways for their desire of becoming-other to flow, in a post-recovery sociality, where there are already expectations in place that contradict the deterritorialisation made possible in the recovery assemblage. The accounts of both service-users and workers show that in this struggle, policy does not operate as an ally, but as a force that blocks and contributes to the reterritorialisation of these flows of desire. Unpacking these forms of reterritorialisation not only produces one more critical account on the implementation of policy, but also demonstrates that the discussion on policy extends beyond the recovery assemblage to the desires of service-users as they try to flow in other socialities. Discussing issues like employment provides an overview of the wider intervention policy attempts to implement. Through a direct link between 'successful' recovery and employability for example, it becomes apparent that *the current focus of policy is not on the recovery process but on the 'recovered' subject*. Recovery is therefore framed as a space expected to produce functional, productive individuals, able to 'return' to society. This way of thinking produces the substance and its consumption as a problem to be 'solved', and neglects all other connections, built and broken, that rendered the becoming with the substance necessary. Throughout this book, I have attempted to unfold how *the present of recovery matters*, and also how staying in this present, *staying with the trouble of recovery* (Haraway, 1988) paves the way for deterritorialisations that extend beyond the recovery assemblage and provide different, more careful ways of thinking about the investment of desire in the assemblages that we inhabit, the connections that we produce, and how these enhance a body's capacity to act.

The question of drugs and recovery is an ethico-political one. The ways in which the connections enhanced in the recovery assemblage desire to extend beyond it, and the ways in which policymaking, as a force attempting to shape *recovered subjects*, breaks these connections, addresses ethico-political issues that transcend the recovery space. The focus of recovery is *not* on physical disengagement from the substance but on engagement with other bodies and forces that expand life possibilities. Service-users, through their narratives, understand wellbeing in ways that extend well beyond the presence or absence of substances in one's body. Wellbeing in their accounts is linked with the establishment of connections that enhance a body's capacity to act, with the understanding of employment not as the process of getting a job, but as a work that leads to the production of something meaningful with others, with the need to slow down, to resist an accelerated mode of life that does not leave space and time for reflection, or for feelings associated with illbeing to be addressed. These are all ethical and political issues, and rendering them visible is an ethically and politically charged practice (de la Bellacasa, 2011: 90). The choice to position desire, the ways it is being enhanced and blocked, in the focus of attention, is also an ethico-political one. The desire of becoming connected, becoming slow, the ways that employment is discussed, are *political imperatives* that concern *all* bodies, not only recovering ones. The desires unfolded by the service-users express a 'desire for the political in an alternative commons' (Berlant, 2011: 225), without 'reentering the normative public sphere' (ibid: 230). Quoting a worker of 18 ano, the work done in the recovery assemblage is political in the sense that it resists the classification of the human condition as a quantitative issue:

> *I always have the feeling that spaces like 18 ano are poles of resistance against the tendency to measure everything based on numbers and percentages, on the money spent and we have to insist that the human*

condition is a qualitative and not quantitative issue, and everyone has to be given the opportunity, even if they don't make it in the end, to benefit from those services, everyone needs to have the opportunity to get help.

The 'political' here does not stand for gestures of heroic action (Berlant, 2011: 259), but for small, everyday gestures as these were accounted for by service-users, inside and beyond the recovery assemblage; the political stands for a desire for belonging, 'a desire for intimacy, sociality, affective solidarity, and happiness' (ibid: 252), and it is this desire for the political that a different 'logic of policy' would be called to enable. When discussing the practices of 'turning up' and 'checking in', Mol's (2008) call for a 'logic of care' rather than a 'logic of choice' was deployed to account for the complexity of one's engagement with the recovery assemblage. I argue here that a shift in the 'logic of policy' is needed; a shift from the *logic of policy as an intervention*, emerging *outside* and being imposed on the space of recovery, to *a logic of policy as practice* that emerges *inside* the recovery assemblage and focuses on enhancing the practices of care in place, and enables the flows of the becoming desires as these extend to other assemblages.

Following this line of thought, policy would have to focus on the recovery assemblage as it stands, stay with the practices of care already in place. The participants of this project, from Liverpool and Athens, have expressed the belief that all treatment and recovery approaches are useful, and constantly shifting goalposts blocks the connections they build slowly and patiently with both the services and the community. Taking these accounts seriously leads to the conclusion that the process of policymaking should not be about making changes, about choosing between treatment approaches and populations that have to be prioritised, and about implementing those choices through the allocation of funding. Conversely, funding needs to be entangled with practices of care becoming in spaces of treatment, whether these are produced by smaller, larger, harm reduction or recovery-focused services, to enhance these practices and to enable the production of new connections that increase life possibilities.

The benefits of the entanglement of funding with specific caring practices already in place, and a rejection of measurement of 'success' based on pre-established criteria would be specific and immediate, as such a shift would signify the liberation of services from meeting targets that do not reflect the actual needs of the drug using population. In the accounts that follow, Genie's founder and the service's manager argue that measuring 'results' and allocating funding based on such an understanding of 'success' leads to the exclusion of the most vulnerable population of drug users, those struggling with mental health issues:

Most people who presented to us with mental health, I'm just assuming, but my experience will tell me probably about 30% of clients who are primary mental health, and yeah, they are more difficult to have a success story on but, that's OK, we'll take that on the chin. There's no way I'm going to say we can't support this person because they're not going to be a good outcome for us.

I don't like it [payment by results],[1] people can cherry pick, I think that excludes people further from services because actually no one's a lost cause and no one's a no-hoper. I think services that operate on that would see people as, oh we can't help them because they're never going to get it. And that would exclude people further. And I don't think it's a good policy to ever have in. Because some people will need support for the rest of their lives maybe, but then how do you get payment on that, because they might always need the service.

Within the current policy context, the accounts of the workers of both Genie and 18 ano, highlight a gap between what is understood as 'success' in policy and in practice:

It was a great success that 18 [ano] managed to stay open, considering that it works with psychotherapy which is non measurable. That's a victory of 18 [ano] and the work done.

Shifting the logic of policy towards a focus on the practices of care already in place, targets this imbalance. Throughout this book I have argued that *unmeasurable practices of care matter*. Immeasurability is not necessarily to be identified with abstract recovery practices that cannot be grasped or talked about. Conversely, my intention has been to make these practices visible. Following the becoming desires of service-users from their first encounter with substances to their hopes and aspirations for encounters beyond the recovery assemblage, it has been revealed how organically developed practices of care enhance a body's capacity to act, not only within the recovery assemblage but also in all other assemblages with which service-users are connected.

This approach does not just challenge how policy is currently applied, but the *logic of policy* overall. The logic of measurable policy shows little trust in the ability of service workers to collectively shift their practices depending on the service-users' needs. Conversely, a logic of policy entangled with practices of care as they develop through the connections enabled in the recovery assemblage, enacts a position of trust towards service-users and workers, as the most appropriate actors to propose and implement change.

This call for a shift of the 'logic of policy' clearly emerges from an empirical engagement with 'good services'. In the introduction my alignment with the specific recovery assemblages I collaborated with was expressed, as well as my intention to use recovery as a platform for the exploration of caring practices, rather than to produce an all-encompassing praise of recovery. When the epistemological framework of care deployed in this book was accounted for, it was acknowledged that 'care' cannot be uncritically deployed as 'good practice'. It also entails a dark side (Martin, Myers and Viseu, 2015) that can carry dominations, as much as 'good' care can carry possibilities. If we abolish all forms of measuring, how then do we account for 'good' and 'bad' caring practices and services?

At the very beginning of the second chapter, the reasons why recovering voices matter were discussed. I specifically referred to the recovering subjectivities' ability to (a) provide an insight to drug using practices that draws on a recently lived experience, reflected upon within a recovery context, (b) account for the *meaning* of drug treatment, the relationships produced and reproduced within it, as well as its limitations and barriers within specific sociopolitical contexts, and (c) produce, through their accounts, knowledge on the societal elements of the *system* of recovery. These assumptions on why and how recovering voices matter were materialised through the accounts of service-users and workers, producing an empirical framework that led to the understanding of care as entangled with desire. Within this framework they provided specific examples of the connections enabled inside and beyond the recovery assemblage, increasing a body's capacity to act.

Some of these accounts reflect findings of studies on drug use and recovery, emerging through different methodological approaches. A longitudinal study conducted in Norway for example (Svendsen et al., 2017), aiming to follow the substance intake of participants for a decade after the completion of the recovery process, reported that going beyond traditional tracking strategies (Robinson et al., 2007) not only improves retention rates, but also contributes to participants' wellbeing. The researchers were contacting participants biweekly through SMS. If their messages remained unanswered for a day, they were then calling them, and if that did not produce any results either, friends and relatives were contacted to advice on how the participant could be reached. In other words, the participant was not treated as a sample, a source of information that could also be retrieved through other ways, but as a subject whose voice matters. This reflects Genie's daily routine of texting and calling the service-users every morning; a practice that strengthened the connection between the service-users and the service, as this mode of 'checking-in' was perceived as a gesture that reaffirmed the workers' commitment to not just 'tick boxes', but actively care for the service-users' wellbeing.

A shift in the logic of policy would require a close examination and expansion of the research already available, accounting for the connections and relationships that contribute to people's wellbeing. The voices and lived experiences of service-users and workers should be positioned as the focus of attention. While 'consumers' participation' in the formation of policies has been a long-standing demand and point of discussion (Brener et al., 2009; Rance and Treloar, 2015; Roberts, 2014; Treloar et al., 2011), it has also been challenged for its enactment and the ways in which consumers' voices are actually valued (Lancaster et al., 2017, Ritter, Lancaster and Diprose, 2018). I am not arguing for the participation of services and their users in the formation of policy as one of the actors involved, but for policy to primarily derive from the experiences of those crafting recovery daily. This is a time consuming and *slow* process. Becoming slow and connected is not a demand that concerns only recovering subjectivities. It extends to all aspects of life, including the ways we do research and policy. A *slow policymaking process* (Stengers, 2018) would enable the voices of those directly involved to be articulated at their own time and in their own terms, unfolding in a way that does not respond to prefabricated questionnaires and assumptions about what is needed, allowing for emerging desires to be expressed and caring practices to be unpacked. It would do justice to 'people's everyday struggles and interpersonal dynamics [as these] exceed experimental and statistical approaches and demand in-depth listening and long-term engagement' (Biehl and Locke, 2010: 318). Ultimately, this is a call for the de-bureaucratisation of policy; one could say an almost 'impossible' task, given that:

> *Policy is, ultimately, a practice of bureaucracy and institutions. And too often we believe that we must engage this practice or be recognized by it in order to achieve the goals we aim for. This is the case for a lot of the early drug user collectives … And many of them succeeded in this. But this very success entailed the eventual failure of the initial project – the collective practice of attuned care. So here we are, responding to this new form of injustice – this biopolitical injustice – born out of a prior political success. And so it goes.*
>
> (Zigon et al. 2022: 5)

However, this inescapable failure of all ethico-political endeavours, is not a call to give up, but to persist. It's a reminder that worldbuilding, as well as the becoming desires of people in recovery, does not have an end point; it's an ongoing practice in its own right. Foregrounding care for the imagining of policy done otherwise, acts as a potentiality time bomb 'within the "system" that open[s] more sites of potentiality for future experimentations with new worlds' (Zigon, 2019: 12).

Finally, returning to the 'meaning' of recovery, the complexity of the term, as well as of the process of recovery has led to its perception as an abstract concept that needs to be rendered graspable through the provision of treatment tools that constrain and measure it (Groshkova, Best and White, 2013). What slips away from such an approach is that it is exactly this so much feared complexity that makes recovery matter. By shifting the attention from the substance to the encounters that shape the experience of drug use and recovery, I have talked about recovery otherwise. Recovery does not happen to the individual, but to the collective (McLeod, 2017). It emerges through a process where an array of human and non-human bodies, forces, affects and relations become active (Duff, 2014a: 94). It becomes possible through collective, caring practices, through new encounters and another investment of desire. It is by default complex, and it is by staying with the trouble (Haraway, 1988) of this complexity of recovery that we can start to imagine another logic of policy, one that aids, rather than obstructs the working of assemblages for health (Andrews and Duff, 2019: 130); one that enhances the organic development of practices of care, enabling deterritorialisations that do not just transform individuals but worlds, inside and beyond the recovery assemblage.

Note

1

> *Payment by results (PbR) is an approach to allocating resources to services that rewards activity or outcomes. Payment depends on what the service does or achieves, for example, on how many hip replacements it performs or how many people it gets into sustainable employment.*

(Roberts, 2011)

For evaluations of the approach see Donmall and Sutton, 2017; Jones et al., 2018; Webster (2017) www.russellwebster.com/final-drug-pbr-report/

References

Advisory Council on the Misuse of Drugs, 1988. *AIDS and drugs misuse (Part 1)*. London: HMSO.

Alacovska, A., 2018. 'Keep hoping, keep going': Towards a hopeful sociology of creative work. *The Sociological Review,* 67(5), pp. 1118–1136.

Allen, R.E. and Wiles, J.L., 2016. A rose by any other name: Participants choosing research pseudonyms. *Qualitative Research in Psychology,* 13(2), pp. 149–165.

Anderson, B., 2006. Becoming and being hopeful: Towards a theory of affect. *Environment and Planning D: Society and Space,* 24(5), pp. 733–752.

Andrews, G.J. and Duff, C., 2019. Matter beginning to matter: On posthumanist understandings of the vital emergence of health. *Social Science & Medicine,* 226, pp. 123–134.

Artaud, A., 1976. *The peyote dance.* Translated by H. Weaver. New York: Farrar, Straus and Giroux.

Askew, R., 2016. Functional fun: Legitimising adult recreational drug use. *International Journal of Drug Policy,* 36, pp. 112–119.

Becker, H.S., 1953. Becoming a marihuana user. *American Journal of Sociology,* 59(3), pp. 235–242.

Berlant, L., 2011. *Cruel optimism.* Durham: Duke University Press.

Berridge, V., 1980. The making of the Rolleston report 1908–1926. *Journal of Drug Issues,* 10(1), pp. 7–28.

Berridge, V., 2012. The rise, fall, and revival of recovery in drug policy. The *Lancet,* 379(9810), pp. 22–23.

Biehl, J. and Locke, P., 2010. Deleuze and the anthropology of becoming. *Current Anthropology,* 51(3), pp. 317–351.

Bignall, S. and Rigney, D., 2019. Transforming colonial systems: Indigeneity, nomad thought and posthumanism. In: Braidotti, R. and Bignall, S., eds., *Posthuman ecologies: Complexity and process after Deleuze.* London: Rowman & Littlefield, pp. 159–181.

Boal, A., 1995. *The rainbow of desire.* Translated by A. Jackson. London: Routledge.

Bøhling, F., 2014. Crowded contexts: On the affective dynamics of alcohol and other drug use in nightlife spaces. *Contemporary Drug Problems,* 41(3), pp. 361–392.

Bøhling, F., 2015. Alcoholic assemblages: Exploring fluid subjects in the night-time economy. *Geoforum,* 58, pp. 132–142.

Bøhling, F., 2017. Psychedelic pleasures: An affective understanding of the joys of tripping. *International Journal of Drug Policy,* 49, pp. 133–143.

Boothroyd, D., 2006. *Cultural on drugs: Narco-cultural studies of high modernity.* Manchester: Manchester University Press.

Bourdieu, P., 1998. *Practical reason: On the theory of action.* Cambridge: Polity Press.

Bourgois, P., 1995. *In search of respect: Selling crack in El Barrio.* Cambridge: Cambridge University Press.

Bourgois, P., 2000. Disciplining addictions: The bio-politics of methadone and heroin in the United States. *Culture, Medicine and Psychiatry,* 24(2), pp. 165–195.

Bourgois, P. and Schonberg, J., 2009. *Righteous dopefiend.* Berkeley: University of California Press.

Brener, L., Resnick, I., Ellard, J., Treloar, C. and Bryant, J., 2009. Exploring the role of consumer participation in drug treatment. *Drug and Alcohol Dependence,* 105(1–2), pp. 172–175.

Bristow, A.B., 2018. Actualising the virtual, *Annual Review of Critical Psychology,* 14, pp. 67–84.

Broekaert, E., 2001. Therapeutic communities for drug users: Description and overview. In: Rawlings, B. and Yates, R., ed., *Therapeutic communities for the treatment of drug users.* London and Philadelphia: Jessica Kingsley Publishers, pp. 29–42.

Campbell, N.D. and Shaw, S.J., 2008. Incitements to discourse: Illicit drugs, harm reduction, and the production of ethnographic subjects. *Cultural Anthropology,* 23(4), pp. 688–717.

Chatwin, C., 2007. Multi-level governance: The way forward for European illicit drug policy? *International Journal of Drug Policy,* 18(6), pp. 494–502.

Clayton, J., Donovan, C. and Merchant, J., 2016. Distancing and limited resourcefulness: Third sector service provision under austerity localism in the north east of England. *Urban Studies,* 53(4), pp. 723–740.

Cohen-Cruz, J., 2012. *Engaging performance: Theatre as call and response.* London: Routledge.

Colebrook, C., 2001. *Gilles Deleuze.* London: Routledge.

Cooper, D.G., 1967. *Psychiatry and anti-psychiatry.* London: Tavistock.

Dahl, S.L., 2015. Remaining a user while cutting down: The relationship between cannabis use and identity. *Drugs: Education, Prevention and Policy,* 22(3), pp. 175–184.

Decorte, T., 2001. Drug users' perceptions of 'controlled' and 'uncontrolled' use. *International Journal of Drug Policy,* 12(4), pp. 297–320.

de la Bellacasa, M.P., 2010. Ethical doings in naturecultures. *Ethics, Place and Environment,* 13(2), pp. 151–169.

de la Bellacasa, M.P., 2011. Matters of care in technoscience: Assembling neglected things. *Social Studies of Science,* 41(1), pp. 85–106.

de la Bellacasa, M.P., 2012. 'Nothing comes without its world': Thinking with care. *The Sociological Review,* 60(2), pp. 197–216.

DeLanda, M., 2016. *Assemblage theory.* Edinburgh: Edinburgh University Press.

Deleuze, G., 1988. *Spinoza: Practical philosophy.* Translated by R. Hurley. San Francisco: City Lights Books.

Deleuze, G., 1990. *The logic of sense.* Translated by M. Lester. London: Athlone Press.

Deleuze, G., 1994. *Difference and repetition.* Translated by P. Patton. London: Athlone Press.

Deleuze, G., 1998. *Essays critical and clinical.* Translated by D.W. Smith and M.A. Greco. London: Verso.

Deleuze, G., 2007. *Two regimes of madness: Texts and interviews 1975–1995.* Translated by A. Hodges and M. Taormina. New York: Semiotext(e).

Deleuze, G. and Guattari, F., 1977. *Anti-Oedipus: Capitalism and schizophrenia.* Translated by R. Hurley, M. Seem and H.R. Lane. New York: Penguin Books.

Deleuze, G. and Guattari, F., 2004. *A thousand plateaus: Capitalism and schizophrenia.* Translated by B. Massumi. London: Continuum.

Dennis, F., 2016. Encountering 'triggers' drug–body–world entanglements of injecting drug use. *Contemporary Drug Problems,* 43(2), pp. 126–141.

Dennis, F., 2019. *Injecting bodies in more-than-human worlds.* London: Routledge.

Dennis, F., Rhodes, T. and Harris, M., 2020. More-than-harm reduction: Engaging with alternative ontologies of 'movement' in UK drug services. *International Journal of Drug Policy,* 82.

Dilkes-Frayne, E., 2014. Tracing the 'event' of drug use: 'Context' and the coproduction of a night out on MDMA. *Contemporary Drug Problems,* 41(3), pp. 445–479.

Dilkes-Frayne, E. and Duff, C., 2017. Tendencies and trajectories: The production of subjectivity in an event of drug consumption. *Environment and Planning D: Society and Space,* 35(5), pp. 951–967.

Donmall, M. and Sutton, M., 2017. *Evaluation of the drugs and alcohol recovery payment by result pilot programme. Final report.* Manchester: University of Manchester.

Duff, C., 2007. Towards a theory of drug use contexts: Space, embodiment and practice. *Addiction Research & Theory,* 15(5), pp. 503–519.

Duff, C., 2011. Networks, resources and agencies: On the character and production of enabling places. *Health & Place,* 17(1), pp. 149–156.

Duff, C., 2014a. *Assemblages of health: Deleuze's empiricism and the ethology of life.* London and New York: Springer.

Duff, C., 2014b. The place and time of drugs. *International Journal of Drug Policy,* 25(3), pp. 633–639.

Duff, C., 2015. Governing drug use otherwise: For an ethics of care. *Journal of Sociology,* 51(1), pp. 81–96.

Duff, C. and Price-Robertson, R., 2018. Deterritorialising the psychological subject (for a 'people to come'). *Annual Review of Critical Psychology – Putting the Deleuzian machine to work in psychology,* 14, pp. 93–110.

Ezzy, D., 2010. Qualitative interviewing as an embodied emotional performance. *Qualitative Inquiry,* 16(3), pp. 163–170.

Farrugia, A., 2015. 'You can't just give your best mate a massive hug every day': Young men, play and MDMA. *Contemporary Drug Problems,* 42(3), pp. 240–256.

Fitzgerald, F.S., 1945. *The crack-up.* New York: New Directions.

Fitzgerald, J., 1998. An assemblage of desire, drugs and techno. *Angelaki: Journal of the Theoretical Humanities,* 3(2), pp. 41–57.

Fitzgerald, J., 2002. Drug photography and harm reduction: Reading John Ranard. *International Journal of Drug Policy,* 13(5), pp. 369–385.

Fitzgerald, J., 2010. Images of the desire for drugs. *Health Sociology Review,* 19(2), pp. 205–217.

Fitzgerald, J., 2015. *Framing drug use: Bodies, space, economy and crime.* London and New York: Springer.

Fomiatti, R., Moore, D. and Fraser, S., 2019. The improvable self: Enacting model citizenship and sociality in research on 'new recovery'. *Addiction Research & Theory*, 27(6), pp. 527–538.

Foot, J., 2015. *The man who closed the asylums: Franco Basaglia and the revolution in mental health care*. London and New York: Verso.

Fotopoulou, M. and Parkes, T., 2017. Family solidarity in the face of stress: Responses to drug use problems in Greece. *Addiction Research & Theory*, 25(4), pp. 326–333.

Foucault, M., 1977. Preface. In: Deleuze, G. and Guattari, F. *Anti-Oedipus: Capitalism and schizophrenia*. New York: Penguin Books, pp. xi–xiv.

Foucault, M., 1986. Of other spaces. Translated by J. Miskowiec. *Diacritics*, 16(1), pp. 22–27.

Foucault, M., 1990. *The history of sexuality: An introduction, volume I*. Translated by R. Hurley. New York: Vintage.

Fox, N.J., 2002. Refracting 'health': Deleuze, Guattari and body-self. *Health*, 6(3), pp. 347–363.

Fox, N.J., 2012. *The body*. Cambridge: Polity Press.

Frank, D., 2018. "I was not sick and I didn't need to recover": Methadone maintenance treatment (MMT) as a refuge from criminalization. *Substance Use & Misuse*, 53(2), pp. 311–322.

Fraser, S., Treloar, C., Bryant, J. and Rhodes, T., 2014. Hepatitis C prevention education needs to be grounded in social relationships. *Drugs: Education, Prevention and Policy*, 21(1), pp. 88–92.

Fraser, S. and valentine, K., 2008. *Substance and substitution: Methadone subjects in liberal societies*. London and New York: Springer.

Garcia, A., 2010. *The pastoral clinic: Addiction and dispossession along the Rio Grande*. Berkeley and Los Angeles: University of California Press.

Garcia, A., 2015. Serenity: Violence, inequality, and recovery on the edge of Mexico City. *Medical Anthropology Quarterly*, 29(4): 1–18.

Genie In the Gutter. [Online]. Available at: www.genieinthegutter.co.uk/home (Accessed 09 December 2019).

Genosko, G., 2009. *Félix Guattari: A critical introduction*. London and New York: Pluto Press.

Giddens, A., 1998. *The third way: The renewal of social democracy*. Cambridge and Malden: Polity Press.

Gill, N., Singleton, V. and Waterton, C., 2017. The politics of policy practices. *The Sociological Review Monographs*, 65(2), pp. 3–19.

Given, L.M., Opryshko, A., Julien, H. and Smith, J., 2011. Photovoice: A participatory method for information science. *Proceedings of the American Society for Information Science and Technology*, 48(1), pp. 1–3.

Glassman, S., Kottsieper, P., Zuckoff, A. and Gosche, E., 2013. Motivational interviewing and recovery: Experiences of hope, meaning, and empowerment. *Advances in Dual Diagnosis*, 6(3), pp. 106–120.

Goat, E., 2015. *ERT: the inside story of Greece's free speech experiment*. [Online]. Available at: www.opendemocracy.net/en/can-europe-make-it/greeces-two-year-blackout-static-suicide-and-new-selfmanagement-model/ (Accessed 02 September 2022).

Gomart, E., 2002. Methadone: Six effects in search of a substance. *Social Studies of Science,* 32(1), pp. 93–135.

Gomart, E., 2004. Surprised by methadone: In praise of drug substitution treatment in a French clinic. *Body & Society,* 10(2–3), pp. 85–110.

Groshkova, T., Best, D. and White, W., 2013. The assessment of recovery capital: Properties and psychometrics of a measure of addiction recovery strengths. *Drug and Alcohol Review,* 32(2), pp. 187–194.

The Guardian, 2013. *Greece shuts down state broadcaster in search for new savings.* [Online]. Available at: www.theguardian.com/world/2013/jun/11/state-broadcaster-ert-shut-down-greece (Accessed 02 September 2022).

Guattari, F., 1984. *Molecular revolution: Psychiatry and politics.* New York: Penguin Books.

Guattari, F., 2015. *From Leros to La Borde.* Translated by E. Kouki. Athens: Koukkida. [published in Greek].

Guattari, F. and Rolnik, S., 2008. *Molecular revolution in Brazil.* Translated by K. Clapshow and B. Holmes. New York: Semiotext(e).

Guillemin, M. and Drew, S., 2010. Questions of process in participant-generated visual methodologies. *Visual Studies,* 25(2), pp. 175–188.

Haraway, D., 1988. Situated knowledges: The science question in feminism and the privilege of partial perspective. *Feminist Studies,* 14(3), pp. 575–599.

Harper, D., 2002. Talking about pictures: A case for photo elicitation. *Visual Studies,* 17(1), pp. 13–26.

Hellman, M., Berridge, V. and Mold, A., 2016. *Concepts of addictive substances and behaviours across time and place.* Oxford: Oxford University Press.

Hetherington, K., 1997. *The badlands of modernity: Heterotopia and social ordering.* London and New York: Routledge.

HM Government, 2010. *Drug strategy 2010. Reducing demand, restricting supply, building recovery: Supporting people to live a drug free life.* London.

HM Government, 2017. *2017 Drug strategy.* London.

HMSO, 1965. *Drug addiction: The second report of the Interdepartmental Committee.* London: Ministry of Health.

Hughes, K., 2007. Migrating identities: The relational constitution of drug use and addiction. *Sociology of Health & Illness,* 29(5), pp. 673–691.

Hunter, D., 2018. *Chav solidarity.* Nottingham.

Hunter, D., 2020. *Tracksuits, traumas and class traitors.* London: Lumpen.

Ifanti, A.A., Argyriou, A.A., Kalofonou, F.H. and Kalofonos, H.P., 2013. Financial crisis and austerity measures in Greece: Their impact on health promotion policies and public health care. *Health Policy,* 113(1–2), pp. 8–12.

Jackson, A.Y. and Mazzei, L.A., 2013. Plugging one text into another: Thinking with theory in qualitative research. *Qualitative Inquiry,* 19(4), pp. 261–271.

James, I.P., 1971. The London heroin epidemic of the 1960's. *Medico-Legal Journal,* 39(1), pp. 17–26.

Javaid, A., 2015. Male rape myths: Understanding and explaining social attitudes surrounding male rape. *Masculinities and Social Change,* 4(3), pp. 270–294.

Johnson, P., 2006. Unravelling Foucault's 'different spaces'. *History of the Human Sciences,* 19(4), pp. 75–90.

Johnson, P., 2013. The geographies of heterotopia. *Geography Compass,* 7(11), pp. 790–803.

Jones, A., Pierce, M., Sutton, M., Mason, T. and Millar, T., 2018. Does paying service providers by results improve recovery outcomes for drug misusers in treatment in England? *Addiction,* 113(2), pp. 279–286.

Keane, H., 2002. *What's wrong with addiction?* Victoria, Australia: Melbourne University Publishing.

Kelly, T.M. and Daley, D.C., 2013. Integrated treatment of substance use and psychiatric disorders. *Social Work in Public Health,* 28(3–4), pp. 388–406.

Kemp, R., 2013. Rock-bottom as an event of truth. *Existential Analysis: Journal of the Society for Existential Analysis,* 24(1), pp. 106–116.

Kentikelenis, A., Karanikolos, M., Reeves, A., McKee, M. and Stuckler, D., 2014. Greece's health crisis: From austerity to denialism. *The Lancet,* 383(9918), pp. 748–753.

Kentikelenis, A. and Papanicolas, I., 2011. Economic crisis, austerity and the Greek public health system. *The European Journal of Public Health,* 22(1), pp. 4–5.

KETHEA, 2019. *Vote for the autonomy of KETHEA therapeutic communities.* [Online]. Available at: www.kethea.gr/en/nea/vote-for-the-autonomy-kethea-ther apeutic-communities/ (Accessed 02 September 2022).

Kirouac, M., Frohe, T. and Witkiewitz, K., 2015. Toward the operationalization and examination of 'hitting bottom' for problematic alcohol use: A literature review. *Alcoholism Treatment Quarterly,* 33(3), pp. 312–327.

Knight, K.R., 2015. *Addicted. pregnant. poor.* Durham and London: Duke University Press.

Kokkevi, A., Loukadakis, M., Plagianakou, S., Politikou, K. and Stefanis, C., 2000. Sharp increase in illicit drug use in Greece: Trends from a general population survey on licit and illicit drug use. *European Addiction Research,* 6(1), pp. 42–49.

Kooyman, M., 2001. The history of therapeutic communities: A view from Europe. In: Rawlings, B. and Yates, R., ed., *Therapeutic communities for the treatment of drug users.* London and Philadelphia: Jessica Kingsley Publishers, pp. 59–78.

Kuehn, K. and Corrigan, T.F., 2013. Hope labor: The role of employment prospects in online social production. *The Political Economy of Communication,* 1(1), pp. 9–25.

Lahman, M.K., Rodriguez, K.L., Moses, L., Griffin, K.M., Mendoza, B.M. and Yacoub, W., 2015. A rose by any other name is still a rose? Problematizing pseudonyms in research. *Qualitative Inquiry,* 21(5), pp. 445–453.

Lancaster, K., 2017. Rethinking recovery. *Addiction,* 112(5), pp. 758–759.

Lancaster, K., Seear, K., Treloar, C. and Ritter, A., 2017. The productive techniques and constitutive effects of 'evidence-based policy' and 'consumer participation' discourses in health policy processes. *Social Science & Medicine,* 176, pp. 60–68.

Latimer, J., 2018a. Afterword: Materialities, care, 'ordinary affects', power and politics. *Sociology of Health and Illness,* 40(2), 379–391.

Latimer, J., 2018b. Repelling neoliberal world-making? How the ageing–dementia relation is reassembling the social. *The Sociological Review,* 66(4), 832–856.

Leontidou, L., 2012. Athens in the Mediterranean 'movement of the piazzas': Spontaneity in material and virtual public spaces. *City,* 16(3), pp. 299–312.

Liebschutz, J., Savetsky, J., Saitz, R., Horton, N.J., Lloyd-Travaglini, C. and Samet, J.H., 2002. The relationship between sexual and physical abuse and substance abuse consequences. *Journal of Substance Abuse Treatment,* 22(3), pp. 121–128.

Lindén, L. and Singleton, V., 2021. Unsettling descriptions: Attending to the potential of things that threaten to undermine care. *Qualitative Research*, 21(3), pp. 426–441.

Lowry, M., 1965. *Under the volcano.* New York: Lippincott.

Maddock, S. and Hallam, S., 2010. *Recovery begins with hope.* London: National School of Government.

Maher, L., 1997. *Sexed work: Gender, race, and resistance in a Brooklyn drug market.* Oxford: Oxford University Press.

Maher, L., 2002. Don't leave us this way: Ethnography and injecting drug use in the age of AIDS. *International Journal of Drug Policy,* 13(4), pp. 311–325.

Malins, P., 2004. Machinic assemblages: Deleuze, Guattari and an ethico-aesthetics of drug use. *Janus Head,* 7(1), pp. 84–104.

Malins, P., 2017. Desiring assemblages: A case for desire over pleasure in critical drug studies. *International Journal of Drug Policy,* 49, pp. 126–132.

Maloutas, T., 2004. Segregation and residential mobility: Spatially entrapped social mobility and its impact on segregation in Athens. *European Urban and Regional Studies,* 11(3), pp. 195–211.

Manton, E., Pennay, A. and Savic, M., 2014. Public drinking, social connection and social capital: A qualitative study. *Addiction Research & Theory,* 22(3), pp. 218–228.

Marlatt, G.A. and Donovan, D.M., 2005. *Relapse prevention: Maintenance strategies in the treatment of addictive behaviors.* New York and London: Guilford Press.

Martin, A., Myers, N. and Viseu, A., 2015. The politics of care in technoscience. *Social Studies of Science,* 45(5), pp. 625–641.

Mars, S., 2003. Heroin addiction care and control: The British System 1916 to 1984. *Journal of the Royal Society of Medicine,* 96(2), pp. 99–100.

Massumi, B., 2002. Navigating movements: An interview with Brian Massumi. In: Zournazi, M., ed., *Hope: New philosophies for change.* Sydney: Pluto Press, pp. 210–243.

Mathis, G.M., Ferrari, J.R., Groh, D.R. and Jason, L.A., 2009. Hope and substance abuse recovery: The impact of agency and pathways within an abstinent communal-living setting. *Journal of Groups in Addiction & Recovery,* 4(1–2), pp. 42–50.

Matsa, K., 2007. *We looked for people and found shadows: The riddle of toxicomania.* Athens: Agra. [published in Greek].

Matsa, K., 2015. Preface. In: Guattari, F., ed., *From Leros to La Borde.* Translated by E. Kouki. Athens: Koukkida. [published in Greek].

Matsa, K., 2018. *Pariahs among pariahs: Addicts and psychopathology.* Athens: Agra. [published in Greek].

McCann, E.J. and Ward, K., 2012. Policy assemblages, mobilities and mutations: Towards a multidisciplinary conversation. *Political Studies Review,* 10(3), pp. 325–332.

McDermott, P., 2005. The great Mersey experiment: The birth of harm reduction. In: Strang, J. and Gossop, M., ed., *Heroin addiction and the British system vol. 1: Origins and evolution.* London and New York: Routledge, pp. 139–156.

McIntosh, J. and McKeganey, N., 2000. Addicts' narratives of recovery from drug use: constructing a non-addict identity. *Social Science & Medicine,* 50(10), pp. 1501–1510.

McKay, J.R., 2017. Making the hard work of recovery more attractive for those with substance use disorders. *Addiction,* 112(5), pp. 751–757.

McKeganey, N., 2007. The challenge to UK drug policy. *Drugs: Education, Prevention and Policy,* 14(6), pp. 559–571.

McLeod, K., 2017. *Wellbeing machine: How health emerges from the assemblages of everyday life.* Durham: Carolina Academic Press.

Measham, F. and Moore, K., 2008. *The criminalisation of intoxication.* Bristol: Policy Press.

Measham, F., Moore, K. and Welch, Z., 2013. *The reorientation towards recovery in UK drug debate, policy and practice: Exploring local stakeholder perspectives.* Lancashire drug and alcohol action team. http://clubresearch.org/wp-content/uploads/2019/08/LDAAT-P4.pdf

Mische, A., 2009. Projects and possibilities: Researching futures in action. *Sociological Forum,* 24(3), pp. 694–704.

Mitcheson, M., Davidson, J., Hawks, D., Hitchens, L. and Malone, S., 1970. Sedative abuse by heroin addicts. *The Lancet,* 295(7647), pp. 606–607.

Mol, A., 2008. *The logic of care: Health and the problem of patient choice.* London and New York: Routledge.

Mold, A., 2004. The 'British System' of heroin addiction treatment and the opening of drug dependence units, 1965–1970. *Social History of Medicine,* 17(3), pp. 501–517.

Mold, A. and Berridge, V., 2007. Crisis and opportunity in drug policy: Changing the direction of British drug services in the 1980s. *Journal of Policy History,* 19(1), pp. 29–48.

Moore, K. and Measham, F., 2006. Reluctant reflexivity, implicit insider knowledge, and the development of club studies. In: Sanders, B., ed., *Drugs, clubs and young people: Sociological and public health perspectives.* London and New York: Routledge (Taylor & Francis), pp. 13–25.

Murphy, M., 2015. Unsettling care: Troubling transnational itineraries of care in feminist health practices. *Social Studies of Science,* 45(5), pp. 717–737.

Neale, J., Finch, E., Marsden, J., Mitcheson, L., Rose, D., Strang, J., Tompkins, C., Wheeler, C. and Wykes, T., 2014. How should we measure addiction recovery? Analysis of service provider perspectives using online Delphi groups. *Drugs: Education, Prevention and Policy,* 21(4), pp. 310–323.

Neale, J. and Kemp, P.A., 2009. Employment and problem drug use. In: Barlow, J., ed., *Substance misuse: The implications of research, policy and practice.* London: Jessica Kingsley, pp. 94–101.

Neale, J., Nettleton, S. and Pickering, L., 2012. *The everyday lives of recovering heroin users.* London: Royal Society of Arts.

Nettleton, S., Neale, J. and Pickering, L., 2013. 'I just want to be normal': An analysis of discourses of normality among recovering heroin users. *Health,* 17(2), pp. 174–190.

Nicholson, H., 2014. *Applied drama: The gift of theatre.* London: Palgrave Macmillan.

Nikolopoulos, G.K., Sypsa, V., Bonovas, S., Paraskevis, D., Malliori-Minerva, M., Hatzakis, A. and Friedman, S.R., 2015. Big events in Greece and HIV infection among people who inject drugs. *Substance Use & Misuse,* 50(7), pp. 825–838.

Noussia, A. and Lyons, M., 2009. Inhabiting spaces of liminality: Migrants in Omonia, Athens. *Journal of Ethnic and Migration Studies,* 35(4), pp. 601–624.

Oksanen, A., 2013. Deleuze and the theory of addiction. *Journal of Psychoactive Drugs,* 45(1), pp. 57–67.

Olievenstein, C., 1977. *Il n'y a pas de drogués heureux. [There are no happy drug users]* Paris: France Loisirs.

O'Malley, P. and Valverde, M., 2004. Pleasure, freedom and drugs: The uses of 'pleasure' in liberal governance of drug and alcohol consumption. *Sociology,* 38(1), pp. 25–42.

Padgett, D.K., Smith, B.T., Derejko, K., Henwood, B.F. and Tiderington, E., 2013. A picture is worth...? Photo elicitation interviewing with formerly homeless adults. *Qualitative Health Research,* 23(11), pp. 1435–1444.

Patton, P., 2000. *Deleuze and the political.* London and New York: Routledge.

Perkins, D., 2008. Improving employment participation for welfare recipients facing personal barriers. *Social Policy and Society,* 7(1), pp. 13–26.

Pessin, A., 2017. *The sociology of Howard S. Becker: Theory with a wide horizon.* Chicago and London: University of Chicago Press.

Price-Robertson, R., Manderson, L. and Duff, C., 2017. Mental ill health, recovery and the family assemblage. *Culture, Medicine, and Psychiatry,* 41(3), pp. 407–430.

Race, K., 2008. The use of pleasure in harm reduction: Perspectives from the history of sexuality. *International Journal of Drug Policy,* 19(5), pp. 417–423.

Race, K., 2017. Thinking with pleasure: Experimenting with drugs and drug research. *International Journal of Drug Policy,* 49, pp. 144–149.

Raimo, S., 2001. Democratic and concept-based therapeutic communities and the development of community therapy. In: Rawlings, B. and Yates, R., ed., *Therapeutic communities for the treatment of drug users.* London and Philadelphia: Jessica Kingsley Publishers, pp. 43–56.

Rance, J. and Treloar, C., 2015. "We are people too": Consumer participation and the potential transformation of therapeutic relations within drug treatment. *International Journal of Drug Policy,* 26(1), pp. 30–36.

Rawlings, B. and Yates, R., ed., 2001. *Therapeutic communities for the treatment of drug users.* London and Philadelphia: Jessica Kingsley Publishers.

Reuter, P. and Stevens, A., 2007. *An analysis of UK drug policy: A monograph prepared for the UK drug policy commission.* London: UK Drug Policy Commission.

Rhodes, T., Bivol, S., Scutelniciuc, O., Hunt, N., Bernays, S. and Busza, J., 2011. Narrating the social relations of initiating injecting drug use: Transitions in self and society. *International Journal of Drug Policy,* 22(6), pp. 445–454.

Ritter, A., Lancaster, K. and Diprose, R., 2018. Improving drug policy: The potential of broader democratic participation. *International Journal of Drug Policy,* 55, pp. 1–7.

Roberts, M., 2011. *By their fruits: Applying payment by results to drug recovery.* London: UK Drug Policy Commission.

Roberts, M., 2014. Making drug policy together: Reflections on evidence, engagement and participation. *International Journal of Drug Policy,* 25(5), pp. 952–956.

Robinson, K.A., Dennison, C.R., Wayman, D.M., Pronovost, P.J. and Needham, D.M., 2007. Systematic review identifies number of strategies important for retaining study participants. *Journal of Clinical Epidemiology,* 60(8), pp. 757–765.

Room, R., 2004. Disabling the public interest: Alcohol strategies and policies for England. *Addiction,* 99(9), pp. 1083–1089.

Ross, S. and Peselow, E., 2012. Co-occurring psychotic and addictive disorders: Neurobiology and diagnosis. *Clinical Neuropharmacology,* 35(5), pp. 235–243.

Schneider, R., Cronkite, R. and Timko, C., 2008. Lifetime physical and sexual abuse and substance use treatment outcomes in men. *Journal of Substance Abuse Treatment,* 35(4), pp. 353–361.

Shinebourne, P. and Smith, J.A., 2010. The communicative power of metaphors: An analysis and interpretation of metaphors in accounts of the experience of addiction. *Psychology and Psychotherapy: Theory, Research and Practice,* 83(1), pp. 59–73.

Singleton, V. and Mee, S., 2017. Critical compassion: Affect, discretion and policy–care relations. *The Sociological Review,* 65(2_suppl), pp. 130–149.

Sir Humphry, D.R., 1926. *Report of the Departmental Committee on Morphine and Heroin Addiction, HMSO.* London: Ministry of Health.

Slater, H., 2013. *On Guattari.* London: Mayday rooms archive.

Spencer, J., Deakin, J., Seddon, T., Ralphs, R. and Boyle, J., 2008. *Getting problem drug users (back) into employment.* London: UK Drug Policy Commission.

Stengers, I., 2002. A 'cosmo-politics'–risk, hope, change. In: Zournazi, M., ed., *Hope: New philosophies for change.* Sydney: Pluto Press, pp. 244–272.

Stengers, I., 2010. *Cosmopolitics I.* Translated by R. Bononno. Minneapolis: University of Minnesota Press.

Stengers, I., 2011. Comparison as a matter of concern. *Common Knowledge,* 17(1), pp. 48–63.

Stengers, I., 2018. *Another science is possible: A manifesto for slow science.* Translated by S. Muecke. Cambridge: Polity Press.

Stimson, G.V., 1983. Views of a sociologist: Drug problems as an everyday part of our society. *British Journal of Addiction,* 78(2), pp. 120–122.

Strang, J. and Gossup, M., 1994. *Heroin addiction and drug policy: The British system.* Oxford: Oxford University Press.

Strathern, M., 2004. *Partial connections.* Walnut Creek: Altamira Press.

Sultan, A. and Duff, C., 2021. Assembling and diversifying social contexts of recovery. *International Journal of Drug Policy,* 87.

Sumnall, H. and Brotherhood, A., 2012. *Social reintegration and employment: Evidence and interventions for drug users in treatment.* Luxembourg City: Publications Office of the European Union.

Svendsen, T.S., Erga, A.H., Hagen, E., McKay, J.R., Njå, A.L.M., Årstad, J. and Nesvåg, S., 2017. How to maintain high retention rates in long-term research on addiction: a case report. *Journal of Social Work Practice in the Addictions,* 17(4), pp. 374–387.

Talking Drugs, 2012. *'Sisa', the drug of the poor.* [Online]. Available at: www.talkingdrugs.org/sisa-the-drug-of-the-poor (Accessed 02 September 2022).

Tapert, S.F., Ozyurt, S.S., Myers, M.G. and Brown, S.A., 2004. Neurocognitive ability in adults coping with alcohol and drug relapse temptations. *The American Journal of Drug and Alcohol Abuse,* 30(2), pp. 445–460.

Theodoropoulou, L., Vitellone, N. and Duff, C., 2022. Practising recovery: New approaches and policy directions. *International Journal of Drug of Drug Policy,* Introduction for the Special Section on 'Practising recovery: New approaches and policy directions' [in press].

Tragakes, E. and Polyzos, N., 1998. The evolution of health care reforms in Greece: Charting a course of change. *The International Journal of Health Planning and Management,* 13(2), pp. 107–130.

Treloar, C., Rance, J., Madden, A. and Liebelt, L., 2011. Evaluation of consumer participation demonstration projects in five Australian drug user treatment facilities: The impact of individual versus organizational stability in determining project progress. *Substance Use & Misuse,* 46(8), pp. 969–979.

Triandafyllidou, A., Gropas, R. and Kouki, H., ed., 2013. *European modernity and the Greek crisis.* New York: Palgrave Macmillan.

Tsili, S., 1995. *Addiction as an ideological stake: The case of Greece.* Athens: National Institute of Social Research. [published in Greek].

Tuck, E., 2009. Suspending damage: A letter to communities. *Harvard Educational Review,* 79(3), pp. 409–428.

Turchik, J. and Edwards, K.M., 2012. Myths about male rape: A literature review. *American Psychological Association,* 13(2), pp. 211–226.

United Nations Office on Drugs and Crime, 2020. Treaties: Drug-related treaties. [Online]. Available at: www.unodc.org/unodc/en/treaties/ (Accessed 13 January 2020).

Vaiou, D., 2010. *Gender, migration and socio-spatial transformations in Southern European cities.* London: Routledge.

Vitellone, N., 2015. Syringe sociology. *The British Journal of Sociology,* 66(2), pp. 373–390.

Vitellone, N., 2017. *Social science of the syringe: A sociology of injecting drug use.* London and New York: Routledge.

Vitellone, N., 2018. Situating the syringe. *International Journal of Drug Policy,* 61, pp. 62–65.

Vitellone, N., 2021. Sociology and the problem of description. *Qualitative Research,* 21(3), pp. 394–408.

Vitellone, N., Theodoropoulou, L. and Manchot, M. 2022. Recovery as a minor practice. *International Journal of Drug Policy* doi.org/10.1016/j.drugpo.2022.103618

Walmsley, I., 2012. Governing the injecting drug user: Beyond needle fixation. *History of the Human Sciences,* 25(4), pp. 90–107.

Webster, R., 2017. *The payment by results drug recovery pilots failed.* [Online]. Available at: www.russellwebster.com/final-drug-pbr-report/ (Accessed 19 January 2020).

White, W.L. and Kelly, J.F., 2010. Recovery management: What if we *really* believed that addiction was a chronic disorder? In: Kelly J. and White W., eds., *Addiction recovery management.* Totowa: Humana Press, pp. 67–84.

Witkiewitz, K. and Marlatt, G.A., 2009. Relapse prevention for alcohol and drug problems: That was Zen, this is Tao. In: Marlatt, G.A. and Witkiewitz, K., ed., *Addictive behaviors: New readings on etiology, prevention, and treatment.* Washington, DC: American Psychological Association, pp. 403–427.

Yates, R., 1992. *If it weren't for the alligators.* Manchester: Lifeline Project.

Yfantis, D., 2017. *Toxicomania through heroin: Drug use in Greece during the interwar.* Athens: Agra. [published in Greek].

Zibbel, J.E., 2004. Can the lunatics actually take over the asylum? Reconfiguring subjectivity and neo-liberal governance in contemporary British drug treatment policy. *International Journal of Drug Policy,* 15(1), pp. 56–65.

Zigon, J., 2011. *"HIV is God's blessing": Rehabilitating morality in neoliberal Russia.* Berkeley and Los Angeles: University of California Press.

Zigon, J., 2019. *A war on people: Drug user politics and a new ethics of community*. Oakland: University of California Press.

Zigon, J., Vitellone, N., Duff, C. and Theodoropoulou, L., 2022. A conversation about recovery and political activism. *International Journal of Drug Policy,* https://doi.org/10.1016/j.drugpo.2022.103614. [in press].

Zontou, Z., 2013. An allegory of addiction recovery: Exploring the performance of Eumenides by Aeschylus, as adapted by 18 ANO theatre group. *Research in Drama Education: The Journal of Applied Theatre and Performance,* 18(3), pp. 261–275.

Index

For Product Safety Concerns and Information please contact our EU
representative GPSR@taylorandfrancis.com
Taylor & Francis Verlag GmbH, Kaufingerstraße 24, 80331 München, Germany